Care of the Dying
A pathway to excellence

Care of the Dying
A pathway to excellence

SECOND EDITION

Edited by

John Ellershaw

Susie Wilkinson

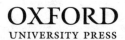

OXFORD
UNIVERSITY PRESS

OXFORD
UNIVERSITY PRESS

Great Clarendon Street, Oxford OX2 6DP

Oxford University Press is a department of the University of Oxford.
It furthers the University's objective of excellence in research, scholarship,
and education by publishing worldwide in

Oxford New York

Auckland Cape Town Dar es Salaam Hong Kong Karachi
Kuala Lumpur Madrid Melbourne Mexico City Nairobi
New Delhi Shanghai Taipei Toronto

With offices in

Argentina Austria Brazil Chile Czech Republic France Greece
Guatemala Hungary Italy Japan Poland Portugal Singapore
South Korea Switzerland Thailand Turkey Ukraine Vietnam

Oxford is a registered trade mark of Oxford University Press
in the UK and in certain other countries

Published in the United States
by Oxford University Press Inc., New York

© Oxford University Press, 2003, 2011

British Library Cataloguing in Publication Data
Data available

Library of Congress Cataloging in Publication Data
Data available

Typeset in Minion by Glyph International, Bangalore, India
Printed in Great Britain
on acid-free paper by
Clays Ltd

ISBN 978–0–19–955083–8

10 9 8 7 6 5 4 3 2 1

Contents

Foreword

Cicely Saunders

'We cannot take away the whole hard thing that is happening, but we can help to bring the burden into manageable proportions.' (1)

The above contribution to a seminar on pain in 1962 was an early attempt to present an approach to the 'total pain' that may be faced by a whole family group as one of its members approaches death. Detailed reports of 900 patients in St Joseph's Hospice where the regular giving of opiates was introduced from 1958 had, by the early 1960s, shown that neither tolerance nor drug dependence need be clinical problems. It was claimed that the end of life could be a time of achievement for both patients and families, leaving the latter with good memories. That such studies should influence both the introduction of specialist research and education centres and be incorporated into the whole health care system, were aims from the beginning.

The challenges presented by the crisis of imminent death are frequently not recognized and patients and families are parted with little opportunity for dealing with unfinished business or making important farewells. The detailed and much quoted USA Support Study showed how common this was in a number of general hospitals, with poor communication and symptom control remaining unaddressed even after a sustained effort to change this unsatisfactory situation (2).

The introduction of specialist multidisciplinary teams to general hospitals started in the 1970s and since then the spread of palliative care world-wide has often begun with such initiatives. The increasing body of research-based knowledge from the special centres, shared with the ward teams, has shown that the earlier they are involved the easier has been the final course of illness, and that changing gear and simplifying therapy to appropriate levels has been less fraught for both staff and family.

In his book 'Death foretold' Christakis has brought together detailed evidence of the difficulty doctors experience in presenting a poor prognosis. He writes, 'the ritualization of optimism, although useful in many respects, can also have negative effects. It may lead physicians and patients to make choices that are ultimately harmful to patients and their families. At its starkest, too much optimism near the end of life may mean patients never see the end coming, never prepare for it, and fight vainly against it.' (3)

If the general ward team, initially with information and support from the palliative care team, can demonstrate that the end of life can be effectively eased, it gives comfort and confidence to all concerned. 'I just want to go off peaceful, like that old lady over there', said a patient interviewed for a hospice video and, 'Efficiency is very comforting', commented a bereaved relative at a day after death meeting.

Much of the now considerable knowledge base has come from the initial concentration on death from cancer but the time has now certainly come for its wider dissemination. 'At the outset of a new initiative it is good practice to establish or pilot a project in a single group and a standard process in health service research. Cancer patients were an identifiable group with suffering and pain.' (4) Justice certainly demands that people dying from any disease in general hospital wards or in the community should reap the benefits of the early work.

The introduction of care pathways has been an example of collaboration across disciplines and directorates. Preparing the ground for such a pathway for care of the dying is an essential part of this process. Sharing expertise with perceptive leadership helps the varied group involved with any one person's care become a confident team ready to assess the priorities of the new situation. Recognizing that the time has come for this change of gear is then easier as a new and still positive goal is established. Crisis can focus minds and initiate change.

The 'total pain' of the end of life (5) has more components than the physical. Emotional, social, and spiritual needs are detailed in the care pathway. Although the patient may seem semi-conscious at this stage, the way care is given can still reach the most hidden places. The knowledge that the most important person is present or is coming can make a difference even at the end. So many patients slip away just when a family member has left after a long vigil, that it seems there must often be some reason for this. Perhaps it is a subconscious holding back on the part of the relative or a desire on the part of the patient to spare the pain of that last moment of letting go. It may be important for staff to talk about this to assuage hampering guilt. The reported presence of a known member of staff at that moment may heal memories.

Spiritual need includes familiar rituals but goes further than that. While words hallowed by centuries of use can seem of sudden and helpful relevance, a wordless presence may be all that is needed to bring a whole life to a moment of dignity beyond physical loss.

All the careful details of the pathway discussed in this book are a salute to the enduring worth of an individual life. Such an ending can help those left behind to pick up the threads of memory and begin to move forward. That this should be easier to achieve, not only in hospices and their home care outreach, but also in general hospitals, community care, and nursing homes, will be the result of this significant book. Its pragmatic and yet holistic approach has come from the specialist palliative care teams and their research and teaching of the past years. Specialist expertise and general challenge meet here in the dimension of our common humanity.

References

1 Saunders C. The treatment of intractable pain in terminal cancer. *Proc R Soc Med*, 1963;**56**:195-7.

2 **The SUPPORT Principal Investigators.** A controlled trial to improve care for seriously ill hospitalised patients. *JAMA*, 1995;**274**:1591-8.

3 Christakis NA. (1999). *Death foretold: Prophecy and prognosis in medical care,* 178. University of Chicago Press, Chicago and London.

4 Wasson K, and George R. (2001). Specialist palliative care for non-cancer patients: The ethical arguments. In *Palliative care for non-cancer patients* (ed. J. M. Addington-Hall and I. J. Higginson), 234–43. Oxford University Press, Oxford.

5 Clark D. Total pain: Disciplinary power and the body in the work of Cicely Saunders 1958–67. *Soc Sci Med*, 1999;**49**:727–36.

Contributors

Maria Bolger
LCP Facilitator, Marie Curie
Palliative Care Institute
Liverpool (MCPCIL), University
of Liverpool, UK

Massimo Costantini
Head, Regional Palliative Care
Network, National Cancer Research
Institute, Genoa, Italy

Andrew Dickman
Senior Clinical Pharmacist
Marie Curie Palliative Care Institute
Liverpool (MCPCIL)
University of Liverpool
UK

Rita Doyle
Palliative Care Nurse Specialist/
Lecturer Practitioner
Directorate of Palliative Care—
Royal Liverpool and Broadgreen
University Hospital, Liverpool, UK

John Ellershaw
Director, Marie Curie Palliative
Care Institute Liverpool (MCPCIL),
University of Liverpool, UK

Steffen Eychmueller
MD, Head Center for Palliative
Care, Cantonal Hospital St.Gallen,
Switzerland

Carl Johan Fürst
Professor/Medical Director,
Stockholms Sjukhem Foundation,
Sweden

Maureen Gambles
Research and Development Lead
Marie Curie Palliative Care
Institute Liverpool (MCPCIL),
University of Liverpool, UK

Eve Garrard
Honorary Research Fellow
Department of Philosophy
University of Manchester, UK

Paul Glare
Chief, Pain & Palliative Care Service,
Department of Medicine,
Memorial Sloan-Kettering Cancer
Center, New York, USA

Margaret Goodman
Senior Lecturer
Research Facilitator in Practice
Coventry University
University Hospitals Coventry
Warwickshire

Grethe Skorpen Iversen
RN (palliative care nurse), Regional
Centre of Excellence for Palliative
Care, Western Norway

Urska Lunder
Palliative Care Clinician
Director, Palliative Care
Development Institute, Slovenia

Stanley Macaden
Retired CEO Bangalore Baptist
Hospital, Bangalore, India

Tamsin McGlinchey
Research Assistant, Marie Curie
Palliative Care Institute Liverpool
(MCPCIL), University of Liverpool,
UK

Theresa MacKenzie
National Liverpool Care Pathway
(LCP) Lead—NZ
Arohanui Hospice, Palmerston
North, New Zealand

Barbara Monroe
CEO, St Christopher's Hospice,
London, UK
International Observatory on
End of Life Care,
Lancaster University
London, UK

Carole Mula
Macmillan Nurse Consultant in
Palliative Care & Professional
Lead Nurse for the Division of
Clinical Support Services
The Christie NHS
Foundation Trust
Macmillan Nurse Consultant in
Palliative Care
Manchester Primary Care Trust

Deborah Murphy
Directorate Manager Palliative Care,
Royal Liverpool and Broadgreen
University Hospital, Associate
Director MCPCIL

Massimiliano Panella
Professor in Public Health,
Amedeo Avogadro University
of Eastern Piemont, Italy
President of the European
Pathway Association

Anita Roberts
Learning and Teaching Lead,
Marie Curie Palliative Care Institute
Liverpool (MCPCIL),
University of Liverpool, UK

Libby Sallnow
Palliative Care Registrar, Barts
and the London NHS Trust, UK

Walter Sermeus
Professor in patient care
management, Catholic University
Leuven, Belgium
Treasurer of the European
Pathway Association

Gustavo de Simone
Medical Director of Pallium
Latinoamerica (NGO)
Founder member of Arg
Asoc of Pall Care

Ruthmarijke Smeding
Senior Educational Consultant,
Marie Curie Palliative Care
Institute Liverpool (MCPCIL),
University of Liverpool, UK

Rev. Prebendary Peter Speck
Researcher and Former Health
Care Chaplain
Honorary Senior Lecturer
(Palliative Care),
Kings College London, UK

Andrew Thorns
Consultant and Honorary Senior
Lecturer in Palliative Medicine
Pilgrims Hospices in East Kent
East Kent NHS Foundation
University Trust
University of Kent, Kent
UK

Vilma Tripodoro
Coordinator of PC Section,
Lanari Institute—Universidad
de Buenos Aires
Past President of Arg Asoc of
Pall Care

Kris Vanhaecht
Postdoctoral research fellow,
Catholic University Leuven,
Belgium
Secretary general of the
European Pathway Association

Lia Van Zuylen
Medical Oncologist/Coordinator
of Palliative Care Team, Erasmus
MC University Hospital, Rotterdam,
The Netherlands

Raymond Voltz
Department of Palliative Medicine,
University Hospital Cologne,
Germany

Susie Wilkinson
Hon. Senior Lecturer Palliative Care
Marie Curie Palliative Care Research
Unit, Department of Mental Health
Sciences, Royal Free & University
College Medical School, London, UK

Ruben van Zelm
Senior consultant, QConsult,
The Netherlands
Secretary of the European
Pathway Association

Introduction

John Ellershaw

The way we care for the dying reflects the kind of society that we have created and live in. The early vision of the pioneers of the hospice movement was to create an environment of care where patients could die a dignified death with support from their carers. They embraced multiprofessional working and recognized that 'journeying with' was sometimes as important as 'problem solving'. The challenge at the start of the 21st century is to extend the vision of the pioneers to all patients in all care settings.

It is recognized that the overall European demographic of dying is changing. It is estimated that 1 703 000 people died of cancer in Europe in 2006 (1), however with new technology and interventions it is currently predicted that cancer mortality will fall by 11% by 2015 (2). At the same time it is recognized that people are living longer, in 2000 the average proportion of the population in 11 European countries who were over the age of 60 was 21% (range 19–24%), the prediction in those same countries for 2020 is 28% (range 22–32%) (3). With older age comes the increased risk of death from chronic co-morbidities, for example heart failure, chronic obstructive pulmonary disease, and renal failure.

At present 58% of deaths in England occur in NHS hospitals, with deaths at home (18%) and in care homes (17%) collectively accounting for around 35% of all deaths. Hospices account for around 4% of deaths, with 3% occurring in other locations (4). Long term projections indicate that if the trend in home death proportions observed over the last five years continues, less than one in ten (9.6%) people will die at home by 2030. Institutional deaths will increase by over 20% from around 440 000 to around 530 000 per annum. People will die increasingly at older ages, with the percentage of deaths amongst those aged 85 and over rising from 32% in 2004 to 44% in 2030 (5). The need to champion the hospice model of excellence for care of the dying and to transfer this model into other health care settings and for non-cancer patients is therefore a priority.

The need to improve care for the dying is further highlighted by a survey of complaints within the NHS, undertaken by the Healthcare Commission which assessed just over 16 000 complaints made about NHS organizations between

July 2004 and July 2006. Approximately half of these related to care given in acute hospitals, no less than 54% of these related in some way to end of life care (6).

The Liverpool Care Pathway for the Dying Patient (LCP) within the Continuous Quality Improvement Programme was developed in the late 1990s, using tried and tested Integrated Care Pathway (ICP) methodology as part of a service improvement programme (7). A project was developed between the specialist palliative care services at the Royal Liverpool and Broadgreen University Hospitals NHS Trust and the Marie Curie Hospice Liverpool, to develop an integrated care pathway (ICP) based on care of the dying within the hospice setting, with the aim to transfer best practice to other settings.

Some 13 years on, The LCP Central Team within the Marie Curie Palliative Care Institute Liverpool (MCPCIL) at the University of Liverpool has devised and published the LCP generic version 12 document following an extensive two year consultation exercise (Appendix 1). The ethos of the LCP generic document has remained unchanged. The LCP generic version 12 has greater clarity in key areas particularly communication, nutrition, and hydration. The responsibility for the use of the LCP generic version 12 document as part of a Continuous Quality Improvement Programme sits within the governance of an organization underpinned by a robust ongoing education and training pro-gramme supported by specialists in palliative care.

As with all clinical guidelines and pathways the LCP aims to support but does not replace clinical judgement. It is important to ensure that patients and relatives understand that the focus of care has changed and that the patient is deemed to be in the last hours or days of life. This requires skilled communica-tion, including recognition of one's own limitations and the need to involve more specialist support where required. Using the LCP appropriately in any environment requires regular assessment and involves continuous reflection, critical decision making, and clinical skill.

The LCP was identified as an example of best practice within the NICE guid-ance for supportive and palliative care (8). In 2006 the government white paper *Our health, our care, our say: a new direction for community services* (9) further reinforced the need to improve the care for dying patients and their families by prioritizing appropriate staff training and recommending the roll out of frameworks like the LCP across the UK via the Department of Health End of Life Care Programme (10,11).

In 2009 a survey, within the NHS, undertaken by the Healthcare Commission highlighted the LCP as a best practice model (12). In addition to the main thrust of the programme spreading nationally, there are 20 countries in Europe and beyond registered with the Institute. In 2010 the European Association for

Palliative Care White Paper on standards and norms for hospice and palliative care in Europe (13) recommended integrated care pathways, such as the LCP, as an educational and quality assurance instrument to improve care of dying patients in settings that are not specialized in palliative care.

Perhaps one of the most significant impacts the LCP has made within the health care system is its influence at managerial, organizational, and national policy levels driving up the quality of care at the bedside. If palliative care is to be incorporated into mainstream health care systems, then demonstrable outcomes of care are essential for quality assurance and commissioning of services. It is possible to extract demonstrable outcomes for care of the dying by analysing performance against the goals on the LCP. This has been demonstrated clearly with two rounds of the National Care of the Dying Audit—Hospitals (NCDAH) in England (14). This major piece of work has enabled the development of a benchmark for care of the dying in the acute hospital sector with associated key performance indicators.

Care of the dying is increasingly becoming a political priority. In order to address this public and policy agenda the challenge is three-fold. First we need to ensure that health care professionals are educated at undergraduate and postgraduate levels in order to give them the skills and confidence to care well for dying patients. Secondly we must continue to strive to improve care of the dying in all care settings where patients die. Thirdly, the further development of a national and international Continuous Quality Improvement Programme for care of the dying across all care settings is a powerful lever to drive up quality of care for the dying irrespective of diagnosis and place of death. The LCP can act as a catalyst in achieving these challenges.

The second edition of *Care of the Dying: A pathway to excellence* includes updated chapters on symptom control, ethical issues, communication skills, bereavement, and spiritual care written by experts in the field which underpin the use of the LCP. The book incorporates the experience we have gained during the development, implementation, and dissemination of the LCP nationally and internationally. We hope that practitioners will find it a useful, practical guide to empower them to care for dying patients to the level of the best. A bad death is no longer acceptable in our society. The time for change is now.

References

1 Ferlay J, Autier P, Boniol M, Heanue M, Colombet M, Boyle P. Estimates of the cancer incidence and mortality in Europe in 2006. *Ann Oncol* 2007;**18**(3):581–92.
2 Levi F, Lucchini F, Negri E, La-Vecchia C. Continuing declines in cancer mortality in the European Union. *Ann Oncol* 2007;**18**(3):593–5.

3 Davies E, Higginson IJ eds. *Palliative care for older people.* World Health Organization Europe, 2004. http://www.euro.who.int/__data/assets/pdf_file/0009/98235/E82933.pdf (Accessed 20 June 2010)

4 National Statistics. *Mortality Statistics. Series DH1 no. 38. Office for National Statistics,* 2005. http://www.statistics.gov.uk/downloads/theme_health/Dh1_38_2005/DH1_No_38.pdf (Accessed 20 March 2010)

5 Gommes B, Higginson IJ. Where people die (1974–2030): Past trends, future projections and implications for care. *Palliat Med* 2008;**22**:33–41

6 Healthcare Commission *Spotlight on Complaints: A report on second–stage complaints about the NHS in England* 2007.

7 Ellershaw JE, Foster A, Murphy D, Shea T, Overill S. Developing an integrated care pathway for the dying patient. *Eur J Palliat Care* 1997;**4**:203–7.

8 National Institute for Health and Clinical Excellance. *Improving supportive and palliative care for adults with cancer* NICE, 2004.

9 Department of Health. *Our health, our care, our say: a new direction for community services.* (2006). http://www.dh.gov.uk/en/Publicationsandstatistics/Publications/PublicationsPolicyAndGuidance/DH_4127453 (Accessed 20 June 2010)

10 Department of Health *End of Life Care Strategy—promoting high quality care for all adults at the end of life.* DH. London 2008.

11 Department of Health *End of Life Care Strategy—Quality markers and measures for end of life care.* DH. London 2009.

12 Healthcare Commission *Spotlight on Complaints: A report on second—stage complaints about the NHS in England* 2009.

13 European Association for Palliative Care (2010) White Paper on standards and norms for hospice and palliative care in Europe: part 2. *Eur J Palliat Care* 2010;**17**(1):22–33.

14 National Care of the Dying Audit—Hospitals summary reports (2008/2009) http://www.mcpcil.org.uk/liverpool-care-pathway/national-care-of-dying-audit.htm (Accessed: 20 June 2010)

Chapter 1

What about care pathways?

Kris Vanhaecht, Massimiliano Panella,
Ruben van Zelm, and Walter Sermeus

Introduction

Porter et al. (1) stated that healthcare should change and that the purpose of healthcare systems is not to minimize costs but to deliver value for patients, which in the long run results in better health per dollar spent. Three principles should guide this change: (i) delivering value to patients, (ii) medical practice should be organized around medical conditions and care cycles, and (iii) results—risk adjusted outcomes and costs—must be measured. With respect to this change, the role of the multidisciplinary team is to focus on the clinical process innovation (CPI) (2). CPIs are central to the ability of organizations to negotiate the challenges of cost containment and quality improvement, yet many CPIs have not met expectations to improve these primary processes (2). Well organized care processes, medical conditions, or care cycles lead to appropriate outcomes if they include a structured context and a well-functioning multidisciplinary team (3).

Patient safety, quality of care, and efficiency of healthcare procedures are international phenomena. In 1991, Brennan et al. (4) concluded that a substantial amount of injury to patients occurs due to healthcare management and that many injuries result from substandard care processes. One of the most cited reports on this topic was published by Kohn and colleagues of the Institute of Medicine (IOM): *To err is human* (5). Later, other authors from all over the world published similar results on adverse events. The first and fundamental ethical principle in healthcare—do no harm—is now being taken seriously by a wide constituency. Five years after the IOM report, in 2004 Altman et al. (6) concluded that many promising efforts have been launched, but the task is far from complete.

Although adverse events are not uncommon in hospitalized patients, they are by no means inevitable (7). Even if a direct relationship is difficult to establish between variations and errors, reducing variations by standardizing clinical processes is an effective tool to minimize the probability of medical errors (5).

Improvement in healthcare requires the active participation of not only the physicians but of all healthcare workers. Recently, Batalden and Davidoff stated, 'Everyone in healthcare really has two jobs when they come to work every day: to do their work and to improve it!' (8).

The pathway history and definition

Healthcare is changing towards more patient focused care. The organization of the care process related to quality, efficiency, and accessibility will be one of the main areas of interest over the next few years for clinicians, healthcare managers, and policy makers. One of the main methods used to (re)organize a care process is the development and implementation of a care pathway. Care pathways, also known as clinical pathways, integrated care pathways, or critical pathways, are used worldwide for a variety of patient groups (9). They originate from industrial processes and were introduced in healthcare in the early 1980s in the United States (10). The development, implementation, and evaluation of clinical pathways represents one of the structured care methodologies next to, for example, guidelines, protocols, and case management. Clinical pathways are nowadays being implemented, as a method for monitoring processes and processing time, in a wide range of healthcare systems, primarily to improve the efficiency of hospital care while maintaining or improving quality. The first systematic use of clinical pathways took place between 1985 and 1987 at the New England Medical Center in Boston (USA) in response to the 1983 introduction of Diagnosis Related Groups (DRGs) (11). Typically, a reference length-of-stay (LOS) and a budget are assigned to each DRG. In the late 1990s, more than 80% of US hospitals used at least some pathways. In the UK, pathways were introduced in the early 1990s (11). Clinical pathways, or integrated care pathways (ICPs) as they are called in the UK, are primarily considered to be tools for designing care processes, implementing clinical governance, streamlining delivered care, improving the quality of clinical care, and ensuring that clinical care is based on the latest research. From the late 1990s towards the beginning of the 21st century, clinical pathways were disseminated all over the world (11,12). Nowadays clinical pathways are used worldwide as one of the tools to structure or design care processes and improve them within the patient-centred care concept. In most countries, the prevalence of pathways is still rather meagre, especially when one considers the idea that the care of 60–80% of patient groups in general hospitals should be suitable for pathway use (12). When developing the pathway for these patient groups, one needs to take the evidence based key interventions, the interdisciplinary teamwork, the patient involvement, and the available resources into account (13). This complexity makes it clear that introducing pathways into an organization and developing, implementing, and evaluating individual pathways is a complex intervention.

Accordingly, the European Pathway Association (EPA) defines a care pathway as:

> A complex intervention for the mutual decision making and organization of predictable care for a well defined group of patients during a well defined period. Defining characteristics of pathways includes: an explicit statement of the goals and key elements of care based on evidence, best practice, and patient expectations; the facilitations of the communication and coordination of roles, and sequencing the activities of the multidisciplinary care team, patients, and their relatives; the documentation, monitoring, and evaluation of variances and outcomes; and the identification of relevant resources (9).

A care pathway is not defined as a document or a tool but as a 'complex intervention' (9,14–17). The Medical Research Council states that complex interventions in healthcare, whether therapeutic or preventative, comprise a number of separate elements which seem essential to the proper functioning of the intervention although the 'active component' of the intervention that is effective, is difficult to specify (15). If we were to consider a randomized controlled trial of a drug versus a placebo as being at the one end of the spectrum, then we might see a comparison of a stroke unit to traditional care as being at the most complex other end of the spectrum. The greater the difficulty in defining precisely what exactly the 'active component' of an intervention is, and how they relate to each other, the greater the likelihood that you are dealing with a complex intervention (15). Pathways show greater similarity to the complexity of stroke units than to the simplicity of giving a single drug. When developing and implementing a care pathway, part of the active ingredients of the complex intervention are the multidisciplinary teamwork, understanding the practical organization of care and the integration of a set of evidence based key interventions and outcomes.

Because of this complexity it becomes clear that pathways are more than only a piece of paper or a file in the patient record (18). Care pathways are a concept to introduce patient focused care, different models of pathways exist, they are a methodology to support the quality and efficiency improvement process and are made operational on different aggregation levels.

Pathways as a concept, model, process, and product

The concept to introduce patient focused care

The goal of care pathways is to introduce and operationalize the patient focused care concept. Although 'patient focused care' can be found in nearly every mission statement of a hospital, rehabilitation centre or primary care organization, it is not always put into practice. The patient focused concept asks for real patient focused care, which means a disease specific orientation and the involvement of patients as real partners (19). More and more hospitals are now changing towards service line organizations where the patient group is a key unit of organization. The Institute of Medicine stated in their publication, *Crossing the Quality Chasm* (2001) (3), one of the first steps to enhance the quality and safety of healthcare organizations:

> Organize and Coordinate Care Around Patient Needs. The primary purpose of identifying priority conditions is to facilitate the organization of care around the patient's perspective and needs rather than, as in the current system, around types of professionals and organizations (3,19).

Degeling describes the relation between medicine, management, and modernization as 'a dance macabre'. He argues that pathways can help in the integration of the different professional groups because in this model the patient group is the central focus (20). Next to this disease specific orientation, seeing patients as real partners will become even more important. 'Every patient is unique, so deal with their needs as they come up and move them onto the next step'. This is one of the traditional rules to provide access to health care as described by Rogers et al. (2008) (21). The new rule will be that every patient is unique, but they share enough in common that care pathways are a useful norm, and patients and clinicians are able to make choices that differ from these pathways as needed (19,21). To protect pathways against this fear and to build patient centred pathways we need to involve patients as real partners in the development process. Wensing and Elwyn (2003) provide an interesting overview of different methods to incorporate patient's views in healthcare (22). Although patient satisfaction questionnaires are one of the most widely used tools, more in depth methods could be suggested for pathway projects. Open interviews with patients and relatives or performing walkthroughs together with a patient or by a clinician as a mystery patient will provide useful information for the pathway development team (19).

Different models of care pathways exist

Care pathways are a model to standardize and follow-up patient focused care. They combine a variety of methods from quality improvement and operational research used in industry and healthcare. When using or translating these methods, two issues are important: the level of predictability of the care process and the level of agreement between the members of the multidisciplinary team (23). Based on these two issues, three different coordination mechanisms can be described: chain models, hub models, and web models (see Figure 1.1) (24).

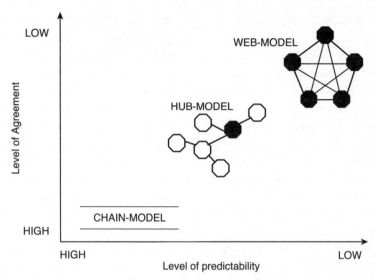

Fig. 1.1 The different models of pathway coordination mechanisms (24).

Chain models are used for high predictability care processes with a high level of agreement between the team members. This mechanism is found for example in elective surgery or chemotherapy processes. For these processes pathways can be used as time-task matrixes, also called Gantt Charts. The sequence of the timing will mostly be day by day. For some more critical care processes, half days or hour by hour will be used to describe the timing of the process.

Hub models are used for less predictable processes like internal medicine, rehabilitation, psychiatry and palliative care. In these models a key person, or case manager, will lead the organization of the care process and can use chain models for the high predictability sub-processes.

Web models are used for unpredictable care or care processes wherein it is necessary to have daily team meetings to be able to organize and structure the process (24). In web models the time-task matrix can be changed into a goal-task matrix. If the time sequence is kept, the day sequence can be changed in weeks. Examples are: complex diagnostic admissions or pathways for patient groups with several important co-morbidities.

One of the goals of each of these models is to enhance the interdisciplinary teamwork (24). The importance of appropriate teamwork cannot be underestimated. Gittel (2000) analysed the relation between good teamwork and patient outcomes and found positive results (25). Vanhaecht et al. found similar results in 2007 (9,26). As already described in a previous section of the chapter (see pathways as a process) the team needs to develop the pathway taking the content and organization into account. Care pathways are, as stated in the definition, interdisciplinary. Different professional groups (doctors, nurses, allied health professionals, etc) need to interact and decide how they will organize the care process and who is responsible and will take the lead for each part. How this challenge is managed will also depend on the level of agreement and predictability as described above (see Figure 1.1).

Chilingerian and Clavin (1994) describe the concept of temporary teams, in which a temporary team is formed for every patient, under the supervision of the clinical lead (medical doctor) and the team members are detached from their own professional group or service (27). When structures are built around these temporary teams and specific resources are invested, the temporary teams may become focused teams (stroke team, total knee team, palliative care team . . .) (28). The interdisciplinary pathway team needs to focus on common goals, describe the different roles of the team members and the communication and coordination mechanisms and processes which will be used. Nelson & Batalden describe clinical microsystems (29). A clinical microsystem is a small, interdependent group of people who work together regularly to provide care for specific groups of patients. This small group is often embedded in a larger organization. Formed around a common purpose or need, these groups may comprise discrete units of care, such as a neonatal intensive care unit or a spine centre. A general clinical microsystem includes, in addition to doctors and nurses, other clinicians, some administrative support and a small population of patients, with information and information technology as critical 'participants' (29). Within a care pathway different clinical microsystems can be defined. The number of people within each microsystem or the number of microsystems within each organization or pathway will differ from organization to organization and model to model (see Figure 1.1) (24).

The quality and efficiency improvement process

Care pathways are also a process on their own to develop and implement well organized care and to improve quality and efficiency (9,18,30). In literature different methodologies are described but basic principles are found in all appropriate methodologies (12,23,31). Active ingredients of the complex care pathway intervention are: the feedback on the actual organization of the care process; the availability of evidence based key interventions and outcome indicators; and the continuous quality and efficiency improvement process which takes place within the multidisciplinary team. Recent multicentre research has shown that during the pathway development, even before the implementation of the pathway, the organization of the care process can be improved (9,26). Over time the team will improve the quality and efficiency of the care process by analysing the actual organization and performance of the care process.

Based on the bottlenecks the team will improve the process by using the plan-do-study-act cycle for continuous improvement with respect to patient characteristics and expectations (9,32). The changes in the organization of the care process are standardized by implementing the pathway product (see Figure 1.2) (9).

To improve the organization, the involvement of the multidisciplinary team will be necessary. Enhancing teamwork is seen as one of the main processes that lead to the improvement of care pathway outcomes. The development of a pathway asks for real teamwork (19). 'Pathways make teams work' is one of the quotes often used during pathway conferences and even in literature. The impact of care pathways on the multidisciplinary teamwork is described in vast amounts of literature but there is a lack of hard evidence on this management issue and it is time to find out what the impact of pathways on teamwork really is. Recently Bates et al. published a list of global priorities in patient safety research (33). When they considered the developed countries, the most important area for research was the lack of coordination and communication, followed by latent organizational failures, poor safety culture, and blame oriented processes (33). A study on the impact of clinical pathways on the organization of care processes (26) revealed that teams who have a pathway to support the care process have significantly higher scores on the coordination of the care process than teams not using pathways (odds ratio 8.92

Clinical/Care Pathway as Continuous Care Process Improvement Intervention

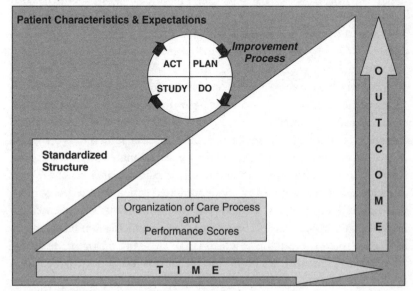

Fig. 1.2 The pathway continuous quality and improvement process (9).

(CI 1.52–95.38) (9,26). Also on the follow-up of the care process a significant odds ratio of 5.56 (CI 1.80–20.36) was found (9). On the overall organization of the care process, measured with the Care Process Self Evaluation Tool (CPSET) (34), a odds ratio of 4.26 (CI 1.40–13.61) in the benefit of pathways was found (9,26). A multicentre study on joint arthroplasty patients, including 39 care processes and 737 consecutive patients, revealed the statistical interaction effect between pathways and the coordination of the care process as determinants for length of stay and elapsed time to discharge (9). Most of these effects are seen in observational studies. Additional research will be necessary to prove the relation between pathways and coordination. The European Pathway Association is currently organizing an international cluster randomized controlled trial on chronic obstructive pulmonary disease and proximal femur fracture patients to explore the impact of pathways on these two patient groups. One of the focuses in these trials is the impact of pathways on the multidisciplinary teamwork (35,36).

One of the most important pitfalls in pathway development from a clinical point of view is the absence or lack of evidence based key interventions and outcome indicators (13,19). During the pathway development process the team needs to review the available literature on the specific clinical topic. Although this can be a very time consuming process it is one of the most important challenges for the future (19). Pathways are used to standardize outcome oriented care, but the content of the pathways is not always clear and is frequently vaguely described in pathway literature. Pathway appraisal instruments describe the development of the pathway, the organization of the care process or the pathway document, but they rarely evaluate the content of the path (18). This problem does not only occur in the field of care pathways but also within the area of clinical guidelines, where the AGREE instrument also does not evaluate the content of the guidelines (37).

One of the possible reasons why some pathways do not lead to an improvement in quality and/or efficiency is the quality of the content. Therefore references to the literature and guidelines should be used in pathways. Websites like *www.guideline.gov* are ideal as a starting point. Google *www.google.com*—although widely used—is not the most appropriate search engine to support evidence based pathways. More evidence based pathways require evidence based key interventions and indicators to follow-up the quality and efficiency. Recently the National Health Service in the United Kingdom has made the *Map of Medicine* available to clinicians. The *Map of Medicine* (*www.mapofmedicine.com*) is a visualization of the ideal, evidence based patient journey for common and important conditions that can be shared across all care settings. The Map is a web-based tool that can help drive clinical consensus to improve quality and safety in any healthcare organization. These Maps, updated every six months, are the start to develop an evidence based pathway. In the Maps the key interventions are described and references to the guidelines and the overall available literature are made available. Pathways can be one of the tools to organize daily clinical practice, based on the evidence based content of the Map.

Next to the Map of Medicine the British Medical Journal Group also provides Action Sets which are detailed overviews of the evidence based content for several care processes. Action Sets from the BMJ Evidence Centre predefine the appropriate diagnostic and treatment orders for a range of common conditions, and can incorporate contextual patient information, local customization and even clinician personalization. They bring critical information from Best Practice, BMJ Point of Care, and Clinical Evidence into the heart of the clinical workflow (*http://group.bmj.com/products/evidence-centre*) (19).

Secondly, evidence based indicators need to be used in the pathways. To develop a pathway is one challenge but to keep pathways alive is a very difficult exercise. To keep pathways alive clinicians, managers, and patients should be frequently provided with hard data on outcomes. A framework for pathway indicators is the Leuven Clinical Pathway Compass in which the five domains are defined: clinical indicators, process indicators, financial indicators, team indicators, and service indicators (38). Pathway facilitators could use the indicator clearing house (comparable to the guideline clearing house) *www. qualitymeasures.ahrq.gov* and the template of the Agency for Healthcare Research and Quality *www.ahrq.gov* to define each indicator. For each indicator the relationship to quality, the benchmark, the definition, the numerator, the denominator, and the type of indicator is described. Also the inclusion and exclusion criteria are important to understand and benchmark the data. Enhancing the level of evidence of the key interventions and outcome indicators should improve the outcome of care. Teams should not forget to include, next to the evidence from literature and clinical research, evidence based on the competence of the team, operational research, and from patient involvement (9,22,24).

The pathway product has four aggregation levels

Next to pathways as a concept, a process, and a method, we have to describe pathways as a product. The pathway product is of course an important item but without the pathway concept, process, and method, the product is worth nothing. This means that buying pathways without translating them and adapting them to the specific organization and team could be unsafe and ineffective. The pathway product is mostly seen as a file in the patient record. Although this patient record is mostly paper-based more and more examples can be found of electronic supported pathways (39). Four types or levels of aggregation or pathway products can be described: the model pathway, the operational pathway, the assigned pathway, the completed pathway. The patient version of the pathway encompasses the operational, assigned, and completed pathways. (24). See Figure 1.3.

The model pathway is the most aggregated level. This pathway is based on the available international and national evidence. It is not organization specific. The operational pathway is the pathway that is developed by a specific organization taking into account the information from the model pathway and the characteristics from the specific organization (available competencies, resources . . .). This pathway is organization specific because of the differences between different organizations. The assigned pathway is the pathway that is used for a specific patient and is the pathway that is based on the operational pathway and adapted to the needs of a specific individual patient. The completed pathway is the path that can be reviewed *ex post facto*, after the discharge of the patient. The difference between the completed pathway and the operational pathway provides information about the variances and the level of compliance to the key interventions in the path (30). Based on this information the pathway can be revised and further improved. A last type of pathway is the patient version of the pathway to inform and involve the patient and family about the process of care. Most of the time the patient version is based on the model and operational pathway (9,13,24).

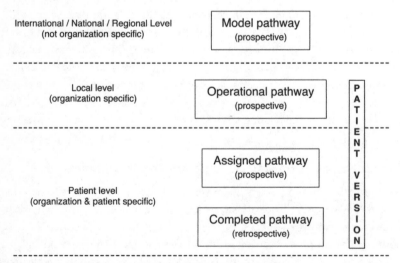

Fig. 1.3 Four aggregation levels of the pathway product (24).

Discussion and challenges for palliative care

Pathways are complex interventions that are more than a piece of paper. They are developed by a multidisciplinary team of clinicians and managers and need to be based on the latest evidence from the literature, operational research, and patient involvement methodologies. Pathways are not something you develop overnight. In palliative care the complex intervention will include the key clinical interventions with a focus on the clinical quality and of course room for caring and supporting activities. The different medical, nursing, spiritual, and allied health professionals need to be part of the development team. Family members should be part of this team and could support the clinicians in the continuous quality and efficiency improvement process.

Pathways need to be developed and implemented with the patient focused care paradigm as the main driver. Different models of pathways can be implemented based on the level of predictability of the care process and the level of agreement within the team. In palliative care a combination of chain, hub, and web models will be found. The model used, will change over time between the palliative diagnosis and the final days, mainly based on the predictability of the process.

Evidence based key interventions and outcome indicators are an important and difficult issue within palliative care. Discussions between the importance of clinical activities or the issue that supporting care is more important will remain a central issue. All interventions in the pathway—clinical, caring, spiritual, supporting, etc—need to be discussed among the different team members so that they lead to shared goals, clear roles, and understandable communication and coordination procedures. Only in this way can the team become a high performance team.

Next to the relation between the professional team and the individual patient, special attention needs to be given to the patient's family. A patient and family version of the pathway, based on the model and operational pathway should be an important by-product for palliative care pathways.

The Liverpool Care Pathway for the Dying Patient (LCP) (40) is a unique example of a model pathway that can be translated and implemented in different organizations all over the world. The work of the Liverpool team, under the supervision and leadership of Professor John Ellershaw, opens up the discussion on how organization specific pathways are. The fact that this pathway is used in different types of organizations, on different continents with different cultures, professionals, competencies, and interests; inspires other clinicians and international networking associations, like the European Pathway Association, to translate this palliative care know-how for other patient groups in different clinical areas. With the development, implementation, and translation of this model pathway for the dying in different cultures and settings, the multidisciplinary team from Liverpool proves that the first and fundamental ethical principle in healthcare—do no harm—must also be taken seriously within the important field of palliative care.

References

1 Porter ME, Olmsted Teisberg E. How physicians can change the future of health care. *JAMA* 2007;**297**(10):1103–11.

2 Savitz LA, Kaluzny AD, Kelly DL. A life cycle model of continuous clinical process innovation. *J Healthcare Man* 2000;**45**(5):307–15.

3 Committee on Quality of Health Care in America IoM. *Crossing The Quality Chasm: A New Health System For The 21st Century*. National Academies Press, Washington DC, 2001.

4 Brennan TA, Leape LL, Laird NM, Hebert L, Localio AR, Lawthers AG, et al. Incidence of adverse events and negligence in hospitalized patients. Results of the Harvard Medical Practice Study I. *N Engl J Med* 1991;**324**(6):370–6.

5 Kohn LT, Corrigan JM, Donaldson MS. *To Err Is Human: Building A Safer Health System*. National Academies Press, Washington DC, 1999.

6 Altman DE, Clancy C, Blendon RJ. Improving patient safety—five years after the IOM report. *N Engl J Med* 2004;**351**(20):2041–3.

7 Leape LL, Lawthers AG, Brennan TA, Johnson WG. Preventing medical injury. *Qual Rev Bull* 1993;**19**(5):144–9.

8 Batalden PB, Davidoff F. What is 'quality improvement' and how can it transform healthcare? *Qual Saf Health Care* 2007;**16**(1):2–3.

9 Vanhaecht K, De Witte K, Sermeus W. *The impact of clinical pathways on the organisation of care processes*. Leuven: ACCO; 2007.

10 Moder JJ, Phillips CF. *Project Management with CPM and PERT*. New York: Reinhold Industrial Engineering and Management Sciences, Textbook Series. Reinhold Publishing Corporation; 1964.

11 Zander K. Integrated Care Pathways: eleven international trends. *J Integrated Care Pathways* 2002;**6**:101–7.

12 Vanhaecht K, Bollmann M, Bower K, Gallagher C, Gardini A, Guezo J, et al. Prevalence and use of clinical pathways in 23 countries - an international survey by the European Pathway Association E-P-A.org. *J Integrated Care Pathways* 2006;**10**:28–34.

13 Vanhaecht K, De Witte K, Sermeus W. The care process organisation triangle: a framework to better understand how clinical pathways work. *J Integrated Care Pathways* 2007;**11**:1–8.

14 Panella M, Marchisio S, Gardini A, Di Stanislao F. A cluster randomized controlled trial of a clinical pathway for hospital treatment of heart failure: study design and population. *BMC Health Serv Res* 2007;**7**:179.

15 Medical Research Council. *A framework for development and evaluation of RCTs for complex interventions to improve health*. Medical Research Council; London 2000.

16 Campbell NC, Murray E, Darbyshire J, Emery J, Farmer A, Griffiths F, et al. Designing and evaluating complex interventions to improve health care. *BMJ* 2007;**334**(7591):455–9.

17 Panella M, Brambilla R, Marchisio S, Di SF. Reducing stroke in-hospital mortality: organized care is a complex intervention. *Stroke* 2008;**39**(11):e186.

18 Vanhaecht K, De Witte K, Depreitere R, Sermeus W. Clinical pathway audit tools: a systematic review. *J Nurs Manag* 2006;**14**(7):529–37.

19 Vanhaecht K, Panella M, Van Zelm RT, Sermeus W. Is there a future for pathways? Five pieces of the puzzle. *Int J Care Pathways* 2009;**13**:82–6.

20 Degeling P, Maxwell S, Kennedy J, Coyle B. Medicine, management, and modernisation: a 'danse macabre'? *BMJ* 2003;**326**(7390):649–52.

21 Rogers H, Maher L, Plsek PE. New design rules for driving innovation in access to secondary care in the NHS. *BMJ* 2008;**337**:a2321.

22 Wensing M, Elwyn G. Methods for incorporating patients' views in health care. *BMJ* 2003;**326**(7394):877–9.

23 Sermeus W, De Bleser L, Depreitere R, De Waele K, Vanhaecht K, Vlayen J. An introduction to clinical pathways. In: Devriese S, Lambert ML, Eyssen M, Van De Sande S, Poelmans J, Van Brabandt H, et al., eds. *The use of clinical pathways and guidelines to determine physicians' hospital fees prospectively: easier said than done.* Brussels: Belgian Healthcare Knowledge Centre (KCE).KCE Reports, Volume 18A, 2005 http://www.kce.fgov.be/index_nl.aspx?SGREF=5270&CREF=5603.

24 Sermeus W, Vanhaecht K. *Van klinische paden naar zorgpaden in Handboek Gezondheidseconomie.* Mechelen: Kluwer; 2009;123–60.

25 Gittell JH, Fairfield KM, Bierbaum B, Head W, Jackson R, Kelly M, et al. Impact of relational coordination on quality of care, postoperative pain and functioning, and length of stay: a nine-hospital study of surgical patients. *Med Care* 2000;**38**(8):807–19.

26 Vanhaecht K, De Witte K, Panella M, Sermeus W. Do pathways lead to better organised care processes? *Journal of Evaluation in Clinical Practice* 2009;**15**:782–8.

27 Chilingerian J, Clavin M. Temporary firms in community hospitals: elements of amanagerial theory of clinical efficiency. *Med Care Review* 1994;**51**(3):289–335.

28 Heskett JL, Sasser J, Earl W, Schlesinger LA. *The service-profit chain: how leading companies link profit and growth to loyalty, satisfaction, and value.* New York: The Free Press; 1997.

29 Nelson EC, Batalden PB, Godfrey MM. *Quality by design: a clinical microsystems approach. Center for the Evaluative Clinical Sciences at Dartmouth.* Jossey-Bass; Wiley, San Francisco 2007.

30 Panella M, Marchisio S, Di SF. Reducing clinical variations with clinical pathways: do pathways work? *Int J Qual Health Care* 2003;**15**(6):509–21.

31 Harkleroad A, Schirf D, Volpe J, Holm MB. Critical pathway development: an integrative literature review. *Am J Occup Ther* 2000;**54**(2):148–54.

32 Deming WE. *Out of the crisis.* Syndicate of the University of Cambridge; Melborne 1982.

33 Bates DW, Larizgoitia I, Prasopa-Plaizier N, Jha AK. Global priorities for patient safety research. *BMJ* 2009;**338**:b1775.

34 Vanhaecht K, De Witte K, Depreitere R, Van Zelm RT, De Bleser L, Proost K, et al. Development and validation of a Care Process Self-Evaluation Tool (CPSET). *Health Services Management Research* 2007;**20**:189–202.

35 Vanhaecht K, Sermeus W, Lodewijckx C, Decramer M, Deneckere S, Leigheb F, et al. *Study Protocol: The European Quality of Care Pathways (EQCP) study on Exacerbation of Chronic Obstructive Pulmonary Disease: a cluster randomized controlled trial* (NCT00962468). European Pathway Association; Leuven: 2009.

36 Vanhaecht K, Sermeus W, Leigheb F, Lodewijckx C, Deneckere S, Peers J, et al. *Study Protocol: The European Quality of Care Pathways (EQCP) study on Proximal Femur Fracture: a cluster randomized controlled trial* (NCT00962910). European Pathway Association; Leuven: 2009.

37 AGREE collaboration. Development and validation of an international appraisal instrument for assessing the quality of clinical practice guidelines: the AGREE project. *Qual Saf Health Care* 2003 Feb;12(1):18–23.

38 Vanhaecht K, Sermeus W. The Leuven Clinical Pathway Compass. *J Integrated Care Pathways* 2003;7:2–7.

39 Rosique R. Do we need electronic support for pathways: the Spanish experience. *International Journal of Care Pathways* 2009;13(2):67–74.

40 Ellershaw JE, Wilkinson SM. *Care of the dying: A pathway to excellence.* Oxford University Press; Oxford 2003.

Chapter 2

What is the Liverpool Care Pathway for the Dying Patient (LCP)?

John Ellershaw and Deborah Murphy

Introduction

The Continuous Quality Improvement Programme of the Liverpool Care Pathway for the Dying Patient (LCP) aims to translate the excellent model of hospice care for the dying into other health care settings and to develop outcome measures using an integrated care pathway (ICP) for the last hours or days of life. The LCP serves to drive up quality whilst improving productivity, and uses innovation to drive and embed change to make a sustainable difference to the way that we care for dying patients and their relatives.

Now, as in the future, a major part of palliative care will be provided by non-specialist services. Consequently, non-specialist professionals must have easy access to specialist consultation for advice and support (1). Integrated care pathways are useful to facilitate and articulate the palliative care approach into a care setting. The LCP is recommended as an educational and quality assurance instrument to improve care of dying patients in settings that are not specialized in palliative care.

The LCP generic document is only as good as the teams using it. Using the LCP generic document in any environment therefore requires regular assessment and involves regular reflection, challenge, critical senior decision making, and clinical skill, in the best interest of the patient. A robust continuous learning and teaching programme must underpin the implementation and dissemination of the LCP generic document. A review of the LCP generic version 11 document began in December 2007 as part of an extensive consultation exercise and the LCP generic version 12 document was published in November 2009.

The LCP Continuous Quality Improvement Programme

Over the past few years a major drive has been underway to ensure that all dying patients, and their relatives or carers receive a high standard of care in the last hours or days of their life. The Liverpool Care Pathway for the Dying Patient (LCP) within the LCP Continuous Quality Improvement Programme is one of the key programmes within the Marie Curie Palliative Care Institute Liverpool (MCPCIL) portfolio.

The LCP Continuous Quality Improvement Programme incorporates:

1 **Aim**

   To improve care of the dying in the last hours or days of life

2 **Key themes**

   To improve the knowledge related to the process of dying

   To improve the quality of care in the last hours or days of life

3 **Key sections**

   Initial assessment

   Ongoing assessment

   Care after death

4 **Key domains of care**

   Physical

   Psychological

   Social

   Spiritual

5 **Key requirements for organizational governance**

   Clinical decision making

   Management and leadership

   Learning and teaching

   Research and development

   Governance and risk

Care in the last hours or days of life

There is an ambiguity regarding the interpretation of terms to articulate the comprehensive care of patients with advanced, incurable life limiting disease. The term end of life care has been used synonymously with the terms palliative care approach, hospice care, care of the dying, and terminal care. It is therefore important to clarify that the LCP generic version 12 document guides and enables healthcare professionals to focus on care in the last hours or days of life. This aims to provide high quality care tailored to the patient's individual needs, when their death is expected. The LCP is designed to be used in the generic environment by generic staff but is best implemented with specialist palliative care support.

Format and outline of the LCP

The LCP document itself has three key sections: initial assessment; ongoing assessment; and care after death, and deals with four primary domains of care: physical, psychological, social, and spiritual. The document consists of a series of goals of care, based on current evidence of 'best practice' that prompt clinicians to focus on the major issues that are likely to be pertinent for patients and their relatives or carers in the last hours or days of life. Information is recorded on the LCP for each of the goals providing an accurate account of the patient's condition and the outcomes of care.

What is variance reporting?

The LCP has the opportunity to record variance. Variance (exception reporting) on an integrated care pathway is a mechanism by which a seemingly process driven approach to care can be tempered in line with individual patient need. The potential to use clinical skill and judgement to deviate from the suggested plan of care in response to an individual patient's needs makes the LCP a more flexible and practical document. Variance recording tells the 'story' of the patient's journey and current condition. Whenever the variance sheets are not completed appropriately, the documentation of care delivery and action required is impoverished.

The appropriate documentation of variance, including information about the issue, the action taken, and the outcome of that action, provides other clinicians involved in the care of the patient with a clear picture of the choices made and the care delivered. Focusing specifically on information documented on the variance sheets allows clinicians to see at a glance what the major issues have been for the patient (and relative or carer) over a given period of time. When variance recording is studied over a cross section of patients, it can also highlight organizational or educational issues that may be impacting on the delivery of care in a given environment. Taking care to document carefully on the variance sheet can, therefore, provide a wealth of important information for clinicians and managers alike. Variance reporting is an important aspect of the process throughout all three sections of the LCP.

Innovation and change model

The implementation of the LCP programme will create a change in the organization. Recognition of the fundamental aspects of a change management programme is pivotal to success. The Service Improvement Model used at the Marie Curie Palliative Care Institute Liverpool (MCPCIL) is a four-phased approach incorporating a 10 step continuous quality improvement process for the LCP programme. See Table 2.1.

A major cultural shift is required if the needs of dying patients are to be met and the workforce are to be empowered to take a leading role in this process. Dying patients are an integral part of the population of our clinical settings. Like any other change within an organization the LCP will require a systematic, coordinated approach to win the hearts and minds of clinicians and to demonstrate the added value to all stakeholders in implementing and sustaining the LCP programme.

Table 2.1 Four phase change management model incorporating a 10 step continuous quality improvement process for the LCP

Phase 1 Induction	STEP 1	Establishing the project—preparing the environment
Phase 2 Implementation	STEP 2	Develop the documentation
	STEP 3	Base review/retrospective audit of current documentation
	STEP 4	Induction/education programme—pilot site
	STEP 5	Clinical implementation of the LCP in pilot sites
Phase 3 Dissemination	STEP 6	Maintaining and improving competencies using reflective practice and post pathway analysis
	STEP 7	Evaluation and further training
	STEP 8	Continuous development of competencies in order to embed the LCP model within the clinical environment
Phase 4 Sustainability	STEP 9	Organizational recognition that all staff who work with people who are dying are properly trained to look after dying patients and their carers within an agreed organizational/educational strategy
	STEP 10	To establish the LCP within the governance/ performance agenda within the organization/ institution

What is organizational governance?

There is no single, comprehensive, universally accepted definition of organizational governance. However, certain common elements are present in most definitions of organizational governance that describe consistent management, cohesive policies, processes, and structures used by an organization to direct and control its activities, achieve its objectives, and protect the interests of its diverse stakeholder groups in a manner consistent with appropriate ethical standards.

Clinical governance is the term used to describe a systematic approach to maintaining and improving the quality of patient care within a health system that embodies three key attributes: recognizably high standards of care, transparent responsibility, and accountability for those standards. The organization strives to continually improve the quality of their services and safeguard high standards of care by creating an environment in which excellence in clinical care will flourish.

LCP generic version 12 document

Following a two year consultation exercise including the latest evidence from two rounds of the National Care of the Dying Audit—Hospitals (NCDAH)(2) (see Chapter 10) the LCP generic version 12 was presented at the sixth annual LCP conference on 25 November 2009, at the Royal Society of Medicine, London, and to the National LCP Reference Group on 2 December 2009; subsequently the LCP core documentation was published on the Marie Curie Palliative Care Institute Liverpool website (see Appendix 1).

The LCP generic version 12 is a single document that supports the care of the patient in the last hours or days of life irrespective of the location of care.

The assessments in Section 2 (ongoing assessment) of the LCP for the community setting (ie patient's own home/residential placement) will be recorded per visit rather than four hourly timed minimal assessments in an inpatient care setting where there is 24 hour trained nursing care (see Appendix 2).

The LCP is only as good as the teams who are using it. As with all clinical guidelines and pathways the LCP aims to support but does not replace clinical judgement. The ethos of the LCP generic document has remained unchanged—LCP generic version 12 has greater clarity in key areas particularly communication, nutrition, and hydration. Care of the dying patient and their relative or carer(s) can be supported effectively by either version of the LCP. The responsibility for the use of the LCP generic document as part of a Continuous Quality Improvement Programme sits within the governance of an organization and must be underpinned by a robust ongoing education and training programme.

Diagnosing dying: the decision to commence the LCP to support care in the last hours or days of life

In order to begin using an LCP to support care, it is essential that clinicians are able to recognize when a patient is dying and has entered the last hours or days of life. The recognition and diagnosis of dying is always complex, irrespective of previous diagnosis or history. Uncertainty is an integral part of the dying process and there are occasions when a patient who was thought to be dying lives longer than expected, and vice versa. For these reasons, clinicians may be reluctant to make a diagnosis that the patient is dying in the hope that the patient's condition may improve. This is particularly so when the prevailing culture is aimed at cure with an associated pressure to continue investigations, invasive procedures, and treatments that may not actually be in the patient's best interest.

LCP generic version 12 includes an algorithm to support the clinical decision making process regarding the recognition and diagnosis of dying and the appropriate use of the LCP to support care in what are thought to be the last hours or days of life (Fig. 2.1). It is important that a diagnosis of dying is made by the multidisciplinary team (MDT). Individual organizations will need to determine the personnel that constitute an MDT, but as a minimum, the MDT will usually be a doctor and nurse but may include other healthcare professionals and personnel as appropriate to a given organization.

The MDT assessment will include the following:

- Is there a potentially reversible cause for the patient's condition? e.g. exclude opioid toxicity, renal failure, hypercalcaemia, infection.
- Could the patient be in the last hours or days of life?
- Is specialist referral needed? e.g. specialist palliative care or a second opinion.

If the patient is diagnosed as dying (in the last hours or days of life) then this should be communicated appropriately. Good, comprehensive, and clear communication is pivotal and all decisions leading to a change in care delivery should be communicated to the patient (where possible and deemed appropriate) and always to the relative or carer. Version 12 of the LCP contains an information sheet which is given to the relatives or carers to support these discussions. The views of all concerned should be listened to and documented, and all subsequent decisions should be documented appropriately on the LCP. If after discussion a consensus is not reached then a second opinion should be sought. Commencement of the LCP requires that health care professionals clearly articulate the date and time of commencement (after a full MDT decision has been made) and that this decision is endorsed (in writing) by the most

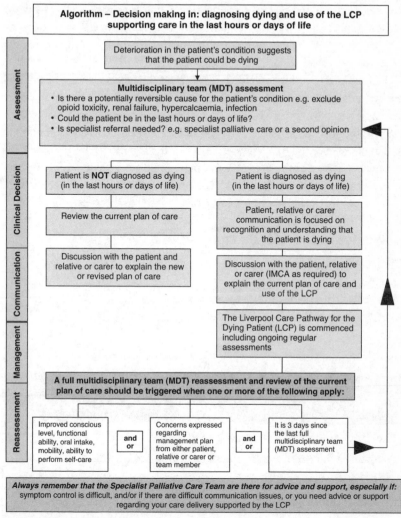

Fig. 2.1 Algorithm: Decision making in—diagnosing dying and the use of LCP supporting care in the last hours or days of life.

senior health care professional who is ultimately responsible for the patient's care at the earliest possible opportunity.

This process should reflect other elements of healthcare clinical decision making. For example, when a decision is made to record a do not attempt cardiopulmonary resuscitation order, this decision must be made by the most senior healthcare professional immediately available in the environment, documented, and witnessed according to local policy and procedure within the organizational governance framework. This decision is then endorsed by the most senior healthcare professional responsible for the patient's care at the earliest opportunity. The LCP generic version 12 calls for the same decision making process to be followed when diagnosing dying and commencing the LCP (see Box 2.1).

Changes in care at this complex and uncertain time should always be made in the best interests of the patient and relative or carer. It is, therefore, important that these needs are reviewed and reassessed regularly whilst the patient is receiving care supported by the LCP, and health care professionals are prompted to undertake regular full MDT reassessments of the situation. These assessments must occur at least every three days but more often where required in response to significant changes in the patient's condition or expressions of concern from relatives or other health care professionals.

How should the LCP be completed?

The following section will take a step by step approach to completing the LCP, providing the rationale for each of the goals of care. Box 2.2 summarizes what health care professionals are expected to do and how to code the LCP accordingly for each of the goals of care. (See Appendix 3 for a completed copy of the LCP.)

Box 2.1 Example documentation from LCP generic version 12 UK document (page 3)

Healthcare professional documenting the MDT decision

Following a full MDT assessment and a decision to use the LCP:

Date LCP commenced:...

Time LCP commenced:...

Name (Print):............................... Signature:.........

This will vary according to circumstances and local governance arrangements. In general this should be the most senior healthcare professional immediately available.

The decision must be endorsed by the most senior healthcare professional responsible for the patient's care at the earliest opportunity if different from above.

Name (Print):............................... Signature:.........

Box 2.2 Section 1: Initial assessment goals (joint assessment by doctor and nurse)

Goal 1.1: The patient is able to take a full and active part in communication

Goal 1.2: The relative or carer is able to take a full and active part in communication

Goal 1.3: The patient is aware that they are dying

Goal 1.4: The relative or carer is aware that the patient is dying

Goal 1.5: The clinical team have up to date contact information for the relative or carer as documented below

Goal 2: The relative or carer has had a full explanation of the facilities available to them and a facilities leaflet has been given

Goal 3.1: The patient is given the opportunity to discuss what is important to them at this time e.g. their wishes, feelings, faith, beliefs, values

Goal 3.2: The relative or carer is given the opportunity to discuss what is important to them at this time e.g. their wishes, feelings, faith, beliefs, values

Goal 4.1: The patient has medication prescribed on a prn basis for all of the following five symptoms which may develop in the last hours or days of life

Pain

Agitation

Respiratory tract secretions

Nausea/vomiting

Dyspnoea

Goal 4.2: Equipment is available for the patient to support a continuous subcutaneous infusion (CSCI) of medication where required

Goal 5.1: The patient's need for current interventions has been reviewed by the MDT

a: Routine blood tests

b: Intravenous antibiotics

c: Blood glucose monitoring

d: Recording of routine vital signs

e: Oxygen therapy

> **Box 2.2 Section 1: Initial assessment goals (joint assessment by doctor and nurse)** (*continued*)
>
> Goal 5.2: The patient has a Do Not Attempt Cardiopulmonary Resuscitation Order in place
>
> Goal 5.3: Implantable cardioverter defibrillator (ICD) is deactivated
>
> Goal 6: The need for clinically assisted (artificial) nutrition is reviewed by the MDT
>
> Goal 7: The need for clinically assisted (artificial) hydration is reviewed by the MDT
>
> Goal 8: The patient's skin integrity is assessed
>
> Goal 9.1: A full explanation of the current plan of care (LCP) is given to the patient
>
> Goal 9.2: A full explanation of the current plan of care (LCP) is given to the relative or carer
>
> Goal 9.3: The LCP Coping with dying leaflet or equivalent is given to the relative or carer
>
> Goal 9.4: The patient's primary health care team/GP is notified that the patient is dying

Section 1: Initial assessment

This assessment should be undertaken by at least a doctor and a nurse. The goals relating to the initial assessment are shown in Box 2.2.

Communication and information: goals 1.1–1.5 and 2

Good, comprehensive, clear communication is an important element in ensuring quality care in the final hours or days of life. The aim is for all patients where possible and relatives or carers to be able to take a full and active part in discussions about the care of the patient and changes to the plan of care in light of the presumed prognosis. All decisions leading to a change in care delivery should be discussed with the patient, wherever possible and deemed appropriate, and with their relatives or carers. It is important that the current level of understanding is explored in order that confidentiality and respect can be maintained in any future discussions that may take place (particularly at the bedside). The views of all concerned should be taken into account and need to be documented carefully.

To do this effectively, health care professionals need to ensure that there are no barriers to communication and to ensure that they have up to date contact details in order that changes in the patient's condition can be communicated sensitively and effectively to the most appropriate person. Information that was accurate at any other time in this episode of care may not be accurate now that the patient is thought to be in the last hours or days of life. In some situations, the next of kin may not be the most appropriate person to contact at the time of impending death and a list of people may be given, or mobile numbers may be needed. Some carers may be working, elderly, or may not wish to be contacted until the following day irrespective of the patient's condition. Establishing how a relative or carer wishes to be told of a patient's impending death is also very important.

Goal 2 is included to ensure that relatives or carers are fully informed about the facilities that are available to them at this point in time. It is important to ensure that this information is given both verbally and in writing, as information given only verbally may not be retained at this sad and challenging time.

Spirituality: goals 3.1 and 3.2

These goals seek to ensure that the patient's and relative's or carer's spiritual needs now, at the time of death, or after death are identified and documented appropriately on the LCP. Opening up a conversation about spiritual beliefs (including religious beliefs) with patients and relatives or carers can enable health care professionals to identify the need for further support from specialist services, as well as providing important information for other health care professionals or personnel who may subsequently become involved with the patient's care. Where it has not been possible to have a conversation directly with the patient, it may be useful to discuss the patient's needs or wishes with the relative or carer.

Medication: goals 4.1 and 4.2

The literature suggests that five main symptoms may develop in the last hours or days of life. Anticipatory prescribing for these five symptoms means minimal delay in responding to a symptom should it arise. It is important to remember, however, that medicines for symptom control should only be given when they are required. The dose should be no more than is needed to control the symptom and should be titrated according to patient needs. For some patients, the use of continuous subcutaneous infusion (CSCI) is indicated and goal 4.2 prompts health care professionals to ensure that this equipment is available as and when required.

Current interventions: goals 5.1–5.3

When the patient is thought to be dying and in the last hours or days of life, it is important that health care professionals review the continued need for interventions and discontinue any that are no longer felt to be conferring benefit. On the other hand, an assessment should be made as to whether any interventions should be commenced in the best interests of the patient at this time. Goal 5.1 prompts health care professionals to consider the following potentially invasive procedures and make decisions based on the best interests of the patient. The need for:

routine blood tests

intravenous antibiotics

blood glucose monitoring

the routine recording of vital signs

oxygen therapy.

Attempting cardiopulmonary resuscitation in patients who have extensive disease and potentially only hours or days to live is generally thought to be futile and inappropriate. Goal 5.2 requires health care professionals to make a decision in the patient's best interests and document appropriately. For the minority of patients who have an implantable cardioverter defibrillator fitted, it is important that this is deactivated according to local policy and with the support of the patient's cardiologist on commencement of the LCP. Goal 5.3 prompts health care professionals to address this issue appropriately where relevant.

Clinically assisted (artificial) nutrition and hydration: goals 6 and 7

The physiological need for food and fluids decreases naturally when the patient is near to death. Whilst patients should be supported to take oral food and fluids for as long as this is tolerated when care is supported by the LCP, health care professionals also need to assess the need for clinically assisted (artificial) nutrition and hydration. As with any clinical guideline or care pathway, the LCP aims to support rather than replace clinical judgement, and health care professionals are asked to stop, think, assess and change practice accordingly. It is important to note that using the LCP does not preclude the use of clinically assisted (artificial) nutrition and hydration, though for many patients this is unlikely to be required. All decisions to discontinue, continue, or commence the use of clinically assisted (artificial) nutrition and hydration must be done in the best interests of each individual patient. The detail of these decisions must then be clearly documented to support the continuity of care.

Skin care: goal 8

Maintaining and promoting the patient's skin integrity (the prevention of the pressure ulcers developing and the prevention of further deterioration of pressure ulcers already present) is an important element in ensuring patient comfort in the final hours or days of life. To this end, Goal 8 encourages health care professionals to develop an appropriate plan of care for each individual patient at this moment in time and to document the plan clearly on the LCP. It is likely that the plan will include regular assessment using recognized risk assessment tools wherever possible, determining the optimum frequency of repositioning and using appropriate aids (special mattresses or beds) where necessary.

Explanation of the plan of care: goals 9.1–9.4

It important to ensure that the patient, wherever possible and deemed appropriate, and the relative or carer are fully aware of the current situation and, more specifically, understand that the plan of care is now focused around maintaining comfort. When engaging in such sensitive discussions, it is important not to assume a level of understanding, but to check how any information you have given has been understood. Goals 9.1 and 9.2 require health care professionals to enter into a dialogue with patients and relatives regarding this issue and to explain the revised plan of care in detail. A leaflet entitled 'Coping with Dying' has been developed specifically to support these conversations and should be given to the relative and carer to take away. The leaflet explains some of the changes in the patient's condition that they might expect as they enter the last hours or days of life and goal 9.3 prompts the appropriate use of this leaflet.

It is important that the patient's primary health care team are also informed about the patient's deteriorating condition and that they are now deemed to be in the last hours or days of life. This is important because the patient, regardless of where they are cared for at the end of their life, remains registered with the primary care practice. Also, GPs in this practice are likely to be responsible for the care of other members of the patient's family who may wish to seek support at this time. It is also important to remember, that even when patients are dying at home and their own GP is involved in care delivery, there may be other members of the healthcare team who may have been providing services until very recently and should be kept fully informed. These may include, the palliative care team, physiotherapy or occupational therapy services, GP receptionist, the chaplaincy team, out of hours services, pharmacist, ambulance services, or the Marie Curie nursing service. Goal 9.4 prompts health care professionals to consider these extended services and notify them as appropriate. (See Appendix 3 for a completed LCP.)

Section 2: Ongoing assessment

The ongoing assessment section (goals a–q in Box 2.3) is where the condition of the patient is monitored on a regular basis for the time that they remain supported by the LCP. Whilst the frequency of monitoring should be determined by patient need, a patient whose care is supported by the LCP must be formally assessed at least every four hours (in inpatient units or where 24 hour nursing care is provided) or at every visit (in the patient's own home). Health care professionals are asked to check the patient and relative or carer's status against the goals of care.

These assessments involve making a judgement at a specific moment in time regarding the level of patient comfort against a series of physical, emotional, and social criteria (goals), and taking appropriate action to improve

Box 2.3 Section 2: Ongoing assessment of the plan of care

Goal a: The patient does not have pain

Goal b: The patient is not agitated

Goal c: The patient does not have respiratory tract secretions

Goal d: The patient does not have nausea

Goal e: The patient is not vomiting

Goal f: The patient is not breathless

Goal g: The patient does not have urinary problems

Goal h: The patient does not have bowel problems

Goal i: The patient does not have other symptoms

Goal j: The patient's comfort & safety regarding the administration of medication is maintained

Goal k: The patient receives fluids to support their individual needs

Goal l: The patient's mouth is moist and clean

Goal m: The patient's skin integrity is maintained

Goal o: The patient receives their care in a physical environment adjusted to support their individual needs

Goal p: The patient's psychological well-being is maintained

Goal q: The well-being of the relative or carer attending the patient is maintained comfort wherever required. Goals of care pertaining to relatives or carers are also included. The outcome of each assessment should be documented carefully on the LCP. Either that the patient is comfortable at the point in time that the assessment is made (coded 'A' for achieved) or that the patient was not comfortable (coded 'V' for variance) and a description of the problem, action taken, and outcome is documented on the appropriate variance sheet.

It is important to remember that these assessments are made of the patient's or relative's or carer's condition at a specific moment in time and not an evaluation of the four hour period since the last assessment (or the period since the last visit). In the inpatient unit, the patient and relative or carer may have been visited several times in the intervening period, and whenever they were found to be in any discomfort (e.g. experiencing pain, agitation and rest-lessness, or emotional distress) appropriate action has been taken and a description of this and the outcome has been documented on the variance sheet. However, this will not be reflected on the four hourly assessment sheet, only on the variance sheet which holds all of the information to enable an in-depth picture over a period of time. Variance reporting is not a negative process, but one that provides a detailed record of the individual nature of the patient's condition based on their particular needs, your clinical judgement, and the ongoing needs of relatives or carers.

Section 3: Care after death

Here the LCP focuses on dignity and respect in the care of the patient's body, the informational needs of relatives or carers in the immediate post bereavement phase (including the provision of bereavement leaflets), and the need to inform other health care professionals involved in the care of the patient and their family of the death of the patient. (See Box 2.4.)

Box 2.4 Section 3: Care after death

Goal 10: Last offices are undertaken according to policy and procedure

Goal 11: The relative or carer can express an understanding of what they will need to do next and are given relevant written information

Goal 12.1: The primary health care team/GP is notified of the patient's death

Goal 12.2: The patient's death is communicated to appropriate services across the organization

Conclusion

A major cultural shift is required if the needs of dying patients are to be met and the workforce are to be empowered to take a leading role in this process. Dying patients are an integral part of the population. Their death must not be considered a failure; the only failure is if a person's death is not as restful and dignified as possible.

Since improvement depends on the actions of people, ultimately it comes down to winning hearts and minds. No matter how good you believe the LCP Continuous Quality Improvement Programme is; you cannot just expect others to do as they are told, nor can you be everywhere at once to ensure compliance. Command and control will not be successful in this process. The LCP is only as good as the teams using it. It represents a step in the right direction towards best practice for all those patients whose death is expected. The LCP document itself will only make a real difference if it is used alongside an implementation and dissemination model firmly embedded in the organization and supported by a continuous learning and teaching programme.

We need to ensure high quality care for our dying patients and their relatives or carers. The quality improvement initiative—quality, innovation, productivity, and prevention (QIPP)(3)—is about creating an environment in which change & improvement can flourish; working and leading differently and in a way that fosters a culture of innovation. It is about providing healthcare professionals with tools, techniques and support that will enable them to take ownership to improve the quality of care given. The LCP is an example of an initiative that captures the hearts and minds of clinicians to respond to and drive the policy agenda, to make a real and lasting difference at the bedside. (See Box 2.5.)

Box 2.5 LCP—Driving up quality of care in the last hours or days of life

Quality: There is only one opportunity to get this right and a good death must become the norm, not the exception in our society.

Innovation: Creating a learning environment where sustainable change comes easily.

Productivity: doing more for less without compromising quality—using limited time and appropriate resources more wisely.

Prevention: Stopping or mitigating problems before they become a crisis.

The LCP can act as a catalyst for organizational change; it can generate discussions on a local, national, and international level that can serve to improve care of the dying from policy to bedside. Although the LCP is recommended as a national and international best practice model for care in the last hours or days of life, success is a journey, not a destination. The road to success is always under construction. We need to continue to build on the evidence base to drive up quality care for all dying patients.

Further resources

National End of Life Care Programme (2010) The route to success in end of life care—achieving quality in acute hospitals, via
http://www.endoflifecareforadults.nhs.uk/assetts/downloads/rts_acute_hospitals.pdf (last accessed 7th July 2010)
General Medical Council(2010) Treatment and care towards the end of life: good practice in decision making—Guidance for doctors, via
http://www.gmc-uk.org/static/documents/content/End_of_life.pdf (last accessed July 2010)

References

1 European Association for Palliative Care White Paper on standards and norms for hospice and palliative care in Europe: part 2. *Eur J Palliat Care* 2010;**17**(1):22–33.
2 National Care of the Dying Audit—Hospitals summary reports (2008/2009) http://www.mcpcil.org.uk/liverpool-care-pathway/national-care-of-dying-audit.htm (accessed 20 June 2010).
3 Department of Health (2010) The NHS Quality, Innovation, Productivity and Prevention Challenge: an Introduction for Clinicians. Department of Health. London.

Chapter 3

Symptom control in care of the dying

Paul Glare, Andrew Dickman, and Margaret Goodman

How can the Liverpool Care Pathway influence symptom control?

The SUPPORT study documented inadequacies in end of life care in American hospitals in the 1990s (1)—inadequacies which were not unique to that time and place, but generalizable to acute care settings in other industrialized countries since the middle of the 20th century. Excellence in end of life symptom control is achieved in hospices but only a small fraction of patients die in a hospice. Specialist palliative care teams have been established in many hospitals to bring hospice principles into acute care, but many patients die without palliative care input, either because the hospital does not have a palliative care service or a consultant from the service is not requested. Integrated care pathways, of which the Liverpool Care Pathway (LCP) is the best known example, take a different approach aiming to effect system-wide change in terminal care.

The LCP was created in the 1990s and has been updated continuously with version 12 published in November 2009 (Appendix 1). The LCP can improve symptom control by providing the generalist hospital staff with an agreed plan of care that specifies goals, guideline-based interventions, and a flow sheet that outlines the expected and realistic course of the patient's care (2,3). Furthermore, each episode can be described, tracked, and monitored to ensure the intermediate and final outcomes for symptom control are within an accepted range of quality. The key components of the LCP are:

1. Identification that the patient is imminently dying, and their care is to be supported by the LCP

2. Initial assessment and care

3. Ongoing assessment

4. Care after death

Importantly, while the LCP provides a useful template to guide the delivery of care it does not replace the skill and expertise of the practitioners using it, both in terms of the decision to commence the LCP and then to recognize and react appropriately to subtle changes in the patients condition. Identifying that a patient is in the last few days of life is relatively straight forward in cancer (4), but may be harder to predict in other eventually fatal illness, e.g. congestive heart failure, chronic obstructive pulmonary disease, or dementia (5). If the LCP is not followed at any point, or a specified goal is not achieved, the health care professional records a reason for the deviation as a 'variance'. An analysis of this variance provides a mechanism for analysing the reasons for not achieving the desired outcomes of the care and helps identify training and resource needs.

Several surveys have indicated that 40–50% patients have uncontrolled pain and other symptoms at the end of life (6–8). Only a small number of evaluations of the LCP have specifically reported impact on symptom control, and have indicated that following the pathway produces much lower rates of symptom problems, but several studies have documented improvements in care that would lead to better symptom control. These include surveying the views of health professionals and carers, and have evaluated the LCP positively (9), including more appropriate use of medications and increased satisfaction with symptom control (10). With regard to the studies documenting actual improvement in symptoms, a study of 168 patients dying on the LCP (53% of all deaths) in the Marie Curie inpatient hospice at Woolton, UK in 1997 found that symptom control (pain, agitation, and respiratory tract secretions) during the last 48 hours of life was achieved for 85% or more of patients. Only 5–10% patients had three or more episodes of uncontrolled symptoms (11). A multi-centre Dutch study, which measured symptom burden in 255 patients cared for on the LCP, found a statistically significant 10–15% reduction in total symptom burden compared to historical controls before the LCP was implemented, with significant reductions in scores for pain, agitation, and troublesome mucus (12).

Other integrated approaches to improving end of life care by generalists in hospitals have been developed in the US, including the Palliative Care for Advanced Disease (PCAD) pathway and order set developed at Beth Israel Medical Center in NY (available at *www.stoppain.org*) and a Comfort Care order set for use by residents at the Mayo Clinic. The PCAD has been shown to lead to an increase in the number of symptoms assessed, although the identification of problematic symptoms and the number of other interventions consistent with the pathway only increased in the inpatient palliative care unit and not on the oncology and geriatric units (13). The Mayo Clinic order set has been shown to significantly improve resident's comfort with ordering medications for symptom management (14).

It needs to be remembered that even in hospitals where an LCP is available not all patients who die will have been supported by the LCP. Despite education staff may not be aware of the LCP, may not accept it, or not be confident in using it. Other patients will deteriorate rapidly or unexpectedly and the LCP would not be used. But, as the pilot testing of the PCAD has shown the system-wide change that results from implementation of an LCP may have a positive flow-on effect to end of life care in general.

What are the commonest symptoms in the dying patient?

Surveys indicate that many symptoms are common at the end of life. Some studies focus on the in-depth characterization of specific symptoms, e.g. delirium (15–17), whereas other reports survey the prevalence of multiple symptoms (6,7,(18–21). A summary of some of these surveys is shown in Table 3.1, and it can be seen that interpreting these data is challenging. Prevalence will depend on the setting and the type of underlying disease, and may change as death gets closer. Some studies distinguish delirium from restlessness and agitation, while others lump them together and include other 'neuropsychological symptoms' such as unconscious and sedation. Similar variations between studies occur with nausea and vomiting; urinary retention and hesitancy; fevers and sweating; myoclonus and seizures. Some studies distinguish background pain and incident pain. Many patients are too ill to report their symptoms; when reported, they are rarely scored for severity. Symptom reports will also be affected by any pharmacological management (22). Reports of the incidence of refractory symptoms would be more helpful when discussing end of life care.

The symptoms of the terminal phase that cause discomfort and need to be addressed are pain, nausea, agitation/restlessness, retained respiratory secretions and breathlessness. Other problems occurring less commonly in the last hours or days of life but impacting on care include inability to swallow, constipation, urinary retention, decubitus ulcers (pressure sores), fever, haemorrhage, seizures, and choking/suffocation. Fortunately, all these symptoms usually only need a handful of medications to be controlled, all of which can be safely given parenterally. There are other terminal symptoms like anorexia and fatigue which are common and not usually considered as requiring treatment, but rather as an accepted and unavoidable part of the dying process.

Table 3.1 Symptom prevalence at end of life

Author	Fainsinger (19)	Conill (21)	Nauck (8)	Lichter (6)	Ellershaw (11)	Grond (11,20)	Goncalves (18)
Year	1991	1997	2001	1990	2001	1991	2003
Setting	Inpatient hospice, Canada	Various palliative care settings, Spain	Palliative care unit, Germany	Inpatient hospice, NZ	Inpatient hospice, UK	Various settings, Germany	Palliative care unit, Portugal
Time before death	1 week	1 week	72 hours	48 hours	48 hours	24 hours	48 hours
% with symptoms							
Pain	99	30	26	51	46	13*	9#
Agitation	-	-	43	42	52	-	-
Delirium	39	68	55	9	-	25	49
Retained secretions	-	-	45	56	45	-	46
Dyspnea	46	47	25	22	-	17	36
Nausea/ vomiting	71	13	14	14	-	10	17
Haemorrhage	-	12	-	-	-	-	15
Seizures	-	-	-	-	-	-	2
Anorexia	-	80	-	-	-	-	
Weakness	-	82	-	-	-	-	
Myoclonic jerking	-	-	-	12	-	-	6
Sweating	-	-	-	14	-	6	31
Urinary problem	-	7	-	53	-	4	8^
Constipation	-	55	-	-	-	12	-
Dysphagia	-	46	-	-	-	9	-
Insomnia	-	-	-	-	-	7	-

*moderate or stronger

#background pain (incident pain 47%)

^urinary retention (urinary incontinence 22%)

How do you manage pain in the dying patient?

Pain control is achievable in the vast majority of patients in the last few days of life using existing methods. Three quarters of dying patients will have pain requiring strong opioid analgesics when they enter the terminal phase. In their final 48 hours, about 13% will then have their dose reduced, 44% will have it increased, and in 48% it will be unchanged (6). One study showed that 60% of patients were able to swallow until they died, 25% needed suppositories, and 15% an injection (23).

More than half will experience a new pain. This may be a new pain problem (e.g. pain control was lost when changing drugs or route of administration; patient has sustained a pathological fracture with handling; oral candidosis is making the mouth and swallowing painful; urinary retention or constipation have developed and not been noticed; pressure ulcers have developed) or else represent escalation of an existing pain due to disease progression. Therefore, even in the dying phase, it is important to keep the four basic principles of pain control in mind (24,25), accepting some modification and adaptation for the dying phase may be required:

1. Identify the noxious stimulus and reverse if possible,

2. Identify and reverse if possible any pain threshold issues

3. When indicated, prescribe opioids

4. If appropriate, prescribe co-analgesic medications

Even in the final hours and days of life, it is important to obtain some pain history and do a focused physical examination. The aim is to identify, if possible, the noxious stimulus causing the pain in case it can be easily eliminated. In patients rapidly approaching the end of life, the use of radiotherapy or invasive analgesic techniques that were indicated earlier in the illness trajectory are usually precluded because the likelihood of relief is small, the burdens and risks are increased, and it is inconvenient to organize outside an acute care setting. Investigations commonly ordered as part of the pain work-up, such as X-rays or neuroimaging, are also not appropriate in the dying phase. It is always important to remember that pain in patients with cancer may not be due to the disease or a side effect of its treatment, but secondary to debility or an unrelated cause. Debility and unrelated causes are more common at this time than earlier in the illness; myofascial pain, constipation, muscle spasm and capsulitis of the shoulder were all debility-related pains making the 'Top 10' pains experienced by patients admitted to Sobell House hospice in an old survey (26).

Pain threshold issues are also likely to be more common at the end of life but may be difficult to assess in the imminently dying patient and may present as terminal agitation/restlessness (see below), rather than articulated as fears and concerns. Psychosocial therapies have limited utility now and pharmacological management with increased doses of opioids and anxiolytics is the mainstay.

In using and increasing the dose of opioids in terminally ill patients, the usual principles of correct prescribing need to be followed. In particular, opioids are not good sedatives and excessive doses will lead to neurotoxicity including delirium and myoclonic jerking (27), which may in turn need treatment (28,29). For patients being cared for with the LCP, there are four opioid prescribing scenarios to consider, determined according to whether or not the patient has pain, and whether or not they are already receiving strong opioids (see Box 3.1). As with patients in earlier stages of the illness, regular review of the level of pain relief is needed and this is prompted by four hourly assessments by the LCP; some experts recommend continuing to monitor pain relief during the dying phase with patient self-report scores (30).

Box 3.1 Four pain scenarios at the end of life

1. Patient is pain free and not on strong opioids. Prescribe subcutaneous morphine 2.5–5 mg four hourly PRN for use if pain develops. This needs to be reviewed after 24 hrs and if more than 2 PRN doses have been given, then a continuous subcutaneous infusion (CSCI) should be considered.

2. Patient is pain free, on strong opioids. Initially the current treatment is continued. If necessary, convert to the subcutaneous route, consider using a CSCI. The patient also needs a rescue dose of morphine prescribed four hourly PRN, for breakthrough pain. This is approximately 1/6th of the 24 hr dose, and would be 2.5–5mg if the patient is receiving 20 mg of morphine over 24 hours via a CSCI. If the patient needs conversion to another strong opioid advice should be sought from a specialist palliative care team.

3. Patient is in pain but opioid naïve. If the pain is constant and moderate to severe in intensity, a strong opioid e.g. morphine (oral or subcutaneous route) 2.5–5mg every 4 hours PRN is used. This needs to be reviewed after 24 hrs and if more than 2 PRN doses have been given, then a CSCI is considered.

4. Patient is in pain and already on oral morphine or other strong opioid. In this situation, current analgesia is ineffective or there is rapidly escalating pain. If the patient does not respond to titration of the opioid dose by 33–50%, or dose limiting toxicity occurs, this constitutes a complex pain problem and a specialist palliative care service should be consulted. Options include opioid rotation or changing route of delivery.

It is usually not recommended to start sustained release oral opioids in the last few days of life, because they may be variable in their absorption and are not suitable for rapid dose titration in patients with uncontrolled pain. But it is reasonable to continue them while the oral route is available, if the pain is controlled. Patient controlled analgesia (PCA) is generally inappropriate, both because the patient may not be able to operate it and, like any equipment at this time, the infusion pump and lines may become a barrier between the patient and family. Indwelling subcutaneous cannulas for intermittent injections or attached to a syringe driver are preferred, as they are small and unobtrusive and are particularly useful in the home where there are visiting nurses trained in their use. Morphine sulphate is the preferred opioid for administration via a continuous subcutaneous infusion (CSCI).

Fentanyl patches now make the transdermal route an obvious alternative to IV or SC in patients who cannot swallow, but there is uncertainty about optimal use of the patches in the dying patient. Like sustained release morphine, patches may be continued in patients whose pain is well controlled, but it is not recommended to initiate them in patients supported by the LCP because of their slow onset of action and difficulty with titration. How one should manage pain which is not well controlled in dying patients on the patches is less clear. It is probably preferable to continue the patch at the same dose and use PRN morphine for rescues in the first 24 hours, then commence a CSCI with morphine sulphate, in addition to the patch, once the 24-hour dose requirement of morphine is clear. In the USA, where hospitalized patients frequently receive IV opioids, normal practice would be to remove the patch and start a fentanyl PCA with stepwise increases in the basal rate during the first 24 hours as the contribution from the residual transdermal dose gradually diminishes. Some analgesic drugs can be given via the rectal route (eg oxycodone suppositories every eight hours) and sublingually (including diamorphine, morphine, phenazocine and dextromoramide) (31) but these routes are less acceptable to some patients, less reliable in terms of absorption, and more limited in terms of drug options and dose ranges.

Incident pain can be a problem in the dying phase. Incident pain is defined as 'a transient exacerbation of pain that occurs either spontaneously or in relation to a specific predictable or unpredictable trigger, experienced by patients who have relatively stable and adequately controlled background pain.'(32) Using this definition, two subtypes of incident pain exist:

- Incident pain—may be predictable (caused by volitional events e.g. when a patient is turned or moved) or unpredictable (caused by involuntary events, such as coughing).

- Spontaneous pain—develops randomly in the absence of a specific trigger

Incident pain can be successfully treated with morphine or alternatively, alfentanil or fentanyl administered via subcutaneous injection.

Correct use of opioids includes education of patient and family to overcome barriers to pain relief (stigma, fear of addiction, side effects). In the dying, there may be an additional fear, that pain relief will hasten death, but this will not occur if proper dose initiation and escalation is applied (33). Management of side effects remains important and patients should continue to take laxatives and antiemetics if needed. In patients with constipation not responding to conventional measures or unable to take oral medications, methylnaltrexone is frequently effective (34). It is contraindicated when there is bowel obstruction.

Adding co-analgesic drugs for components of the pain that are not very opioid responsive demands due consideration of pharmacokinetics, polypharmacy, drug interactions, and side effects, including anticholinergic load (35). As many of these drugs take days to become effective (e.g. gabapentin, tricyclic antidepressants), it would be uncommon to initiate them in the terminal phase, but pre-existing prescriptions may be continued while tolerated. Most of these drugs are problematic in patients who cannot swallow; only a few of these drugs have parenteral formulations (e.g. dexamethasone, ketorolac, clonazepam, ketamine), while some agents from these classes may be available transdermally (e.g. diclofenac, lidocaine) or rectally (e.g. paracetamol, naproxen). On account of their long half lives and the reduction in drug clearance in the final days, antidepressants and anticonvulsants will continue to work for several days after being stopped. Neuropathic pain may respond to a higher dose of opioid. For patients with severe uncontrollable pain and distress sedation may be required (see below). Non-pharmacological management will help many pains occurring in the final few days of life, such as xerostomia (mouth care), decubitus ulcers (mattress changes) and constipation (enemas).

How do you manage agitation in the dying patient?

The presence of restlessness and agitation during the dying phase is a sad and distressing problem. The dissolution of autonomy and dignity associated with an agitated delirium, the associated stigma of mental illness, and the evaporation of quality of life demand quick, active, and aggressive multidisciplinary interventions (36). As with pain and other symptoms, the cause of agitation needs to be identified and reversed if possible, although it is often multifactorial. A precise, potentially reversible aetiology cannot be identified in more than 50% of cases. As with pain and any other symptom in the dying, assessment relies on history taking and the clinical examination, rather than the results of investigations. A single venepuncture to check electrolytes, calcium, glucose, and white cell count could be justified as it is low burden; but it will be done more often for diagnostic reasons than therapeutic ones.

The commonest causes of agitation in the last days of life include drug toxicity (including opioid neurotoxicity), metabolic upset, physical discomfort and anxiety/anguish. If opioid toxicity is suspected, opioid reduction or switching (with or without rehydration) can be tried (29), although the outcome may be difficult to evaluate in such a short time frame. Drug withdrawal from alcohol or benzodiazepines needs to be considered and treated. Metabolic derangement can be corrected although hyper- or hypoglycaemia are probably the only ones where treatment is indicated in the final hours or days of life. Hypoxia can respond to supplementary oxygen. Antibiotics may occasionally be warranted if there is infection causing discomfort that cannot be easily palliated otherwise, or steroids if there are symptomatic brain metastases. Physical discomforts are an important source of agitation/confusion that can be easily remedied: a distended bladder due to urinary retention is very distressing and insertion of a urinary catheter is instantly effective. Similarly, evacuating a distended rectum relieves distress quickly. In a patient with anxiety and or emotional distress, talking should always be tried before medications.

Three clinical forms of delirium have been described: hyperactive, hypoactive, and mixed (37). Patients with hyperactive delirium present with agitation, restlessness, and hallucinations. Hypoactive delirium is commonly confused with depression or medication-related sedation and it is the most frequently observed subtype of delirium. From all patients with delirium, 86% have the characteristics of the hypoactive subtype (38).

There are two main pharmacological approaches in the palliation of agitation: benzodiazepines to provide sedation and antipsychotic drugs to provide tranquilization. In the dying phase, benzodiazepines are usually employed because they are the mainstay of treatment for anxiety or emotional distress and the initial management of confusion (major tranquilizers like haloperidol or levomepromazine have less of a place than prior to the onset of dying phase).

Benzodiazepines are considered to be first line agents for treatment of delirium associated with seizures and alcohol withdrawal. They are frequently used in conjunction with haloperidol in agitated patients. The sedative properties of benzodiazepines can be used in refractory cases requiring sedation. Studies report that up to 30% of terminally ill patients have delirium resistant to treatment with antipsychotics (16,39–42).

Various short- and long-acting benzodiazepines are available, but in the dying phase midazolam is commonly prescribed, via a CSCI (5–20 mg/day initially, titrate up to 30 mg/day or more), or by intermittent injection.

The medication to be prescribed depends on the whether or not the patient is already agitated: if the patient is not currently confused agitated or distressed, a PRN dose of midazolam (2.5–5 mg) subcutaneously four hourly is prescribed. Review the medication usage after 24 hours and if two or more doses have been given then consider a syringe driver, continuing PRN doses accordingly. If symptoms persist, the palliative care team should be consulted. For the management of confusion due to drug toxicity, metabolic derangement, or altered sensorium, a major tranquilizer such as haloperidol or levomepromazine would usually be indicated. Benzodiazepines like midazolam occasionally cause paradoxical behaviour reactions.

Haloperidol is usually preferred to phenothiazines because of its superior side effect profile but levomepromazine or chlorpromazine have both been found to be safe and effective in the dying phase in palliative care (43). Haloperidol has proven its efficacy and relatively safe profile. It is available for administration via different routes. Studies have shown that the typical antipsychotics remain under-utilized and only 17% of terminally ill patients with delirium receive them (37). Starting doses of haloperidol are in the range of 0.5 to 5 mg given orally, intravenously, or subcutaneously (1–2 mg boluses every 30 minutes to one hour, until the patient settles) with total daily dose rarely exceeding 20mg. The total amount given can then be administered as a maintenance dose over 24 hours, either in divided doses or continuously via a CSCI.

In severe cases of agitated delirium, haloperidol is used in conjunction with midazolam, or in the USA, lorazepam. The addition of the benzodiazepine also provides sedation and counteracts the extrapyramidal side effects of haloperidol. Chlorpromazine or levomepromazine are more sedating than haloperidol, so can be administered as a single agent or in combination with a benzodiazepine. Phenothiazines cause hypotension and lower the seizure threshold.

The new generation atypical neuroleptics; risperidone, olanzapine, quetiapine, and ziprasidone are reported to have less extrapyramidal side effects, although it is only at doses of more than 4.5 mg/day of haloperidol that there is an increased rate of side effects in comparison to the atypical antipsychotics (44). Atypical antipsychotics may have a role in severe cases refractory to typical antipsychotics but well designed studies confirming their superiority remain to be conducted. For intractable delirium, palliative sedation may be the only effective therapeutic intervention (36,45). Barbiturates such as phenobarbital and general anaesthetics like propofol may be required as second-line agent for palliative sedation. Uncontrolled pain should always be considered as a possible cause of refractory agitation in a dying patient. While opioids are poor sedatives and neurotoxicity needs to be avoided, increasing the dose of analgesics should always be tried in refractory cases.

In the non-pharmacological management of delirium, a safe environment needs to be provided. Psychological interventions may be helpful, depending on the patient's level of consciousness. Continuity of carers and the presence of a near relative are the most important psychosocial therapeutic strategies (36). Bladder distension in a setting of urinary retention is very distressing and insertion of a Foley catheter is very effective. Similarly, treatment of severe constipation can alleviate delirium.

How do you manage nausea and vomiting in the dying patient?

Nausea and vomiting are unpleasant symptoms and prompt action to control them is essential. A thorough assessment and history is vital in order to identify the cause(s) so as to enable the most suitable choice of anti-emetic. However, this is not always possible. In cases where a cause cannot be identified, the use of a broad-spectrum anti-emetic is suggested. In the UK, either cyclizine or levomepromazine can be considered.

Cyclizine is an antihistamine that exhibits additional anticholinergic activity. These properties give the drug its broad anti-emetic action, with the main action sited within the vomiting centre. In cases of large-volume vomiting due to bowel obstruction, cyclizine may be combined with glycopyrronium (anticholinergic) or octreotide (anti-secretor). Cyclizine occasionally crystallizes with hyoscine butylbromide, so this combination should be avoided. Any mixtures containing cyclizine must be diluted with Water for Injections to prevent incompatibilities. Unwanted effects of cyclizine include drowsiness and dry mouth. Cyclizine should be avoided in severe congestive heart failure and it may occasionally cause irritation at the infusion site.

Levomepromazine is an effective anti-emetic with strong sedative effects as doses increase. It is a particularly useful drug because its pharmacology renders it active at most of the key receptor targets in the vomiting pathway. Some centres do not use levomepromazine first line because of its principal adverse effect of sedation. This is used beneficially, though, in terminal restlessness or agitation (see below). It may cause infusion site reactions, although dilution with sodium chloride 0.9% can overcome this. Levomepromazine can be mixed with all drugs shown in Table 3.2.

Metoclopramide and haloperidol are dopamine antagonists. They are particularly useful if nausea and vomiting is due to drugs or a homeostatic disorder (e.g. renal failure, hypercalcaemia). In addition, metoclopramide is

Table 3.2 Principal drugs for administration via CSCI

Analgesic	Diamorphine Morphine Oxycodone Dose depends upon prior use.	
Anti-emetic	Cyclizine	100–150mg daily
	Metoclopramide	30–60mg daily
	Levomepromazine	6.25–25mg daily
	Haloperidol	5–10mg daily
Sedative	Midazolam	10–100mg daily
	Levomepromazine	25–200mg daily
	Haloperidol	5–10mg daily
Anticholinergic	Glycopyrronium	0.6–2.4mg
	Hyoscine butylbromide	60–180mg
	Hyoscine hydrobromide	0.8–2.4mg

prokinetic and is useful if gastric stasis is believed to be the cause of nausea and vomiting.

How do you manage respiratory tract secretions in the dying patient?

Patients approaching the terminal stages of life are often unable to clear upper respiratory tract secretion which leads to the condition known as the 'death rattle.' In clinical practice, this is a frequently encountered symptom, occurring in up to 92% of dying patients (46). The management of respiratory tract secretions in the dying patient is primarily aimed at minimizing the distress of relatives or carers, rather than the patient. Clinical experience would suggest that most patients are unconscious when terminal secretions are present and it is believed that the patient does not unduly suffer with this symptom. However, there is no evidence to support this and terminal secretions may contribute to the development of dyspnoea and terminal restlessness. The use of parenteral fluids for hydration is not believed to be associated with a worsening of terminal secretions (47).

Treatment of this condition can involve positional changes and pharmacological intervention; difficult cases may require suction. Not all patients will be suitable for positional changes, which involve moving to a position so as to facilitate drainage. Suction is unpleasant and the patient should receive a subcutaneous dose of midazolam (2.5–5mg) prior to the procedure. The main treatment of terminal secretions, therefore, involves the anticholinergic drugs.

Table 3.3 Anticholinergic drug comparisons

	Hyoscine hydrobromide	Glycopyrronium	Hyoscine butylbromide
Ampoule size	400µg/ml	600µg/3ml	20mg/ml
Cost (per ampoule)[†]	£2.88	£1.01	£0.22
Usual daily dose range	1.2–2.4mg	0.6–1.2mg	60–120mg
Daily cost	£8.64–£17.28	£1.01–£2.02	£0.66–£1.32

[†] National Health Service (UK) prices (November 2009)

One important point to remember about these drugs is that they will not remove secretions that are already present. Treatment must be started as soon as symptoms become apparent. Three anticholinergic drugs are available in the UK to treat respiratory tract secretions: hyoscine hydrobromide, glycopyrronium, and hyoscine butylbromide (see Table 3.3). It is surprising that given the relatively common nature of this symptom, there is a paucity of evidence to support the superiority of any of these drugs. A recent randomized trial (48) confirmed the non-superiority of hyoscine butylbromide or hyoscine hydrobromide while a non-randomized study concluded there was no difference in response to hyoscine hydrobromide or glycopyrronium (49). In fact, a review in 2008 concluded that, 'there is currently no evidence to show that any intervention, be it pharmacological or non-pharmacological, is superior to placebo in the treatment of death rattle'. (50) Nonetheless, glycopyrronium is almost one-and-a-half times as potent as hyoscine hydrobromide in preventing salivary secretions, a component of terminal secretions (51). Glycopyrronium is less expensive than hyoscine hydrobromide and is the drug of choice in many centres. Hyoscine butylbromide is the least expensive of the three, but its use in terminal secretions is not as widespread.

Both glycopyrronium and hyoscine butylbromide are quaternary ammonium compounds. This means that neither penetrates the blood brain barrier easily due to the bulky size. Consequently, these drugs are devoid of the sedative and direct anti-emetic effects associated with hyoscine hydrobromide. All three drugs may be administered via a continuous subcutaneous infusion (CSCI) and subcutaneous injections may be given. Hyoscine hydrobromide can be administered via a transdermal patch and has been nebulized to treat terminal secretions (52) but its use in this manner cannot be recommended. For doses and costs of these drugs, refer to Table 3.3.

How do you manage dyspnoea in the dying patient?

Like pain, dyspnoea is a subjective experience involving several factors that influence the degree and perception. As the patient enters the terminal phase it may not be possible or practical to address all of these causes. The aim of treatment changes to focus on the perception of breathlessness and any associated anxiety, ensuring the patient remains comfortable.

Pharmacological intervention forms the mainstay of treatment, although non-drug measures, such as a cool air or a calming hand, may still have a role. Typical pharmacological regimens involve opioids and benzodiazepines. Consideration may also be given to anticholinergic drugs and phenothiazines. As the patient becomes progressively weaker, oral administration of medication may no longer be possible and drugs are commonly given via the subcutaneous route. The rectal route can be used, although suitable preparations do not exist for all drugs. A recent review failed to demonstrate a consistent effect of oxygen in the relief of dyspnoea due to end stage malignancy (53). If the patient is unconscious, consideration to discontinue this treatment can be made. Patients with dyspnoea typically experience tachypnoea and anxiety. It is believed that by reducing the respiratory rate and addressing the associated anxiety, the perception of breathlessness is also reduced.

The opioids act in a variety of ways; essentially they can reduce the respiratory rate and reduce the level of anxiety. Diamorphine, morphine or oxycodone can be administered via subcutaneous injection or infusion. The dose used depends upon previous oral requirements, although for an opioid naïve patient a suitable starting dose would be 10mg of morphine daily. If the patient has been receiving opioids for pain, the dose can be increased to achieve the necessary reduction in respiratory rate to an arbitrary level of 15 breaths per minute. Nebulized morphine has been used in the palliative treatment of dyspnoea with varying results. Until more positive evidence is forthcoming, this route of administration cannot be recommended.

Oral promethazine may also be considered as a second-line agent if systemic opioids cannot be used or in addition to systemic opioids (54). Promethazine should not be administered by subcutaneous injection, but an alternative phenothiazine, levomepromazine, can be considered. There is no evidence to support or disprove its use, but levomepromazine is anxiolytic and may be considered for the treatment of dyspnoea associated with anxiety or agitation. A suitable starting dose would be 12.5mg daily via subcutaneous injection or infusion.

Benzodiazepines may be a useful treatment for patients with dyspnoea associated with anxiety, although a recent review concludes that there is no evidence to recommend the use of benzodiazepines to treat dyspnoea (54). Should a benzodiazepine be considered, midazolam via subcutaneous injection or infusion would be the drug of choice. Stat doses of 2.5–5mg may be given and a continuous infusion titrated according to need. Occasionally, lorazepam is given sublingually at a dose of 0.5–1 mg up to four times daily.

Terminal secretions may contribute to the development of terminal dyspnoea, although evidence is lacking. Nonetheless, an anticholinergic drug, such as glycopyrronium, should be started as soon as terminal secretions become apparent. No patient should believe that they will die suffering from dyspnoea. Although opioids and sedatives are employed, the aim of treatment is to reduce the level of anxiety and improve the sensation of breathlessness, whilst maintaining the patient's level of consciousness. However, this may not always be possible; indeed as the patient becomes weaker, drowsiness becomes more apparent. This should be explained clearly to the patient and their relatives or carers.

What are the benefits of using a continuous subcutaneous infusion (CSCI) to deliver medication?

The last decade has seen several developments in infusion technology. In addition to the Smiths Medical (formerly Graseby) MS16A and MS26, there are three newer devices that are capable of delivering a CSCI: CME McKinley T34, Micrel MP Daily and Cardinal Alaris AD. The syringe driver or pump is a portable battery-operated device that can be used to deliver a continuous subcutaneous infusion. The administration of drugs via a CSCI has been shown to be common practice within specialist palliative care units across the UK and Eire (55). However, the use of CSCIs is not solely limited to palliative care; they have been used successfully in a variety of conditions, such as thalassaemia, myasthenia gravis, and Parkinson's disease.

The condition of an advanced cancer patient is likely to deteriorate, such that parenteral administration of drugs may become necessary. Regular intramuscular or subcutaneous injections are painful; the rectal route is not always appropriate or acceptable; and intravenous injections needlessly increase the risk of infection. The use of a CSCI to deliver drugs allows improved symptom control with less discomfort and inconvenience. A CSCI is often suggested to treat the last few days of life, although it is not restricted to this indication. A single CSCI containing up to four, possibly five, drugs will control the vast majority of symptoms that a dying patient is likely to experience.

The main indications for a CSCI are shown in Box 3.2. A CSCI is extremely beneficial in the hospital, hospice, and home setting and the advantages are shown in Box 3.3. The need to deliver drugs via a CSCI could be for a variety of reasons that do not always mean the end of life is approaching, a fact that should be explained to anxious patients or relatives; it is vital that the patient

Box 3.2 Indications for a CSCI

Oral:	nausea and vomiting
	dysphagia
	severe weakness
	patient preference
	unconsciousness
Rectal:	diarrhoea
	bowel obstruction
	patient preference
IV/IM:	cachexia
	fear

and family are involved because this method of drug administration can be incorrectly associated with dying and hastening death.

It is important that users become familiar with the type of syringe driver or pump that has been adopted in their area of practice as there are clear important differences. For example, the CME McKinley T34 calculates the rate of delivery (in ml/hour) automatically once the syringe is attached and correctly identified; the delivery rate of the MS26 has to be manually entered and is determined by the length of fluid in the syringe per unit time (mm/day) rather than volume. All devices can accommodate a variety of syringe sizes although it is generally recommended for the majority of CSCIs that a 20ml syringe is used (in order to reduce the risk of site reactions and reduce the amount of drug lost in the dead space of the giving set).

Box 3.3 Advantages of a CSCI

Increased patient comfort

Control of multiple symptoms with a combination of drugs

Plasma drug concentrations are maintained without peaks and troughs

Independence and mobility maintained because the device is lightweight and can be worn in a holster either under or over clothes

Generally needs to be assembled only once every 24 hours.

What drugs can be used in a syringe driver?

As the patient approaches the terminal stages of life, it is important to review all medication. A pharmacist can provide useful advice regarding drugs that can be safely discontinued and help with the development of a new treatment strategy. Drugs previously considered essential e.g. cardiac drugs and oral hypoglycaemics, should be reviewed with the intention of discontinuing them. Several treatments can be continued via a CSCI. Indeed, a recent study found that as many as 29 different drugs were being administered via CSCI in adult specialist palliative care units throughout the UK and Eire (55). Nonetheless, most symptoms that a patient is likely to experience during the terminal phase can be adequately controlled with a combination of up to four or five drugs administered via a CSCI (see Table 3.2).

Analgesics

Diamorphine, morphine sulphate and oxycodone are the opioids typically used for CSCIs. Diamorphine is preferred when analgesic requirements are particularly large because it has a significantly greater solubility in water; 1g of diamorphine dissolves in only 1.6ml of water, compared with 21ml for the equivalent amount of morphine sulphate. The dose to administer depends upon previous opioid requirements, but for an opioid naïve patient, a suitable dose would be 5–10mg morphine/oxycodone over 24 hours. Common opioid conversion factors are shown in Table 3.4. Note that equianalgesic doses are difficult to determine and initial dose conversions should be conservative. Aim for the lowest equianalgesic dose if a range is stated; it is safer to under-dose the patient and use rescue medication for any shortfalls. Should the patient be

Table 3.4 Equianalgesic factors of common opioids (Adapted from reference 56)

Opioid	Conversion factor to subcutaneous morphine or oxycodone* (mg)
Codeine (oral)	0.05
Diamorphine (sc)	1.5
Fentanyl (72 hour transdermal dose)	See text
Hydromorphone (oral)	3.75
Morphine (oral)	0.5
Oxycodone (oral)	0.5–0.66

* Based on a 1:1 conversion between subcutaneous morphine and oxycodone.

To calculate the dose, multiply the dose of opioid (in milligrams) by the conversion factor. For example, 120mg oxycodone (oral) x 0.66 = 80mg oxycodone (sc)

Table 3.5 Determination of practical rescue doses of subcutaneous opioids for patients using a fentanyl patch

Fentanyl patch strength	Diamorphine rescue dose	Morphine/Oxycodone rescue dose
12μg/hour	2.5mg	5mg
25μg/hour	5mg	10mg
50μg/hour	10mg	15mg
75μg/hour	15mg	20mg
100μg/hour	20mg	30mg

currently using a fentanyl patch, it would be sensible to continue with this. Rescue doses of subcutaneous diamorphine, morphine or oxycodone should be given to treat poorly controlled background pain. Refer to Table 3.5 to determine suitable rescue doses. After 24 hours, the total number of rescue doses should be totalled and administered via a CSCI, in addition to the fentanyl patch.

> For example: Consider a patient currently prescribed a fentanyl 50μg/hour patch. This is considered equivalent to 90mg of subcutaneous morphine. The rescue dose of morphine via subcutaneous injection would be 15mg. If the patient required two rescue doses in a 24 hour period, 30mg of morphine would then be added to a CSCI. This is in addition to the patch. The new rescue dose would be 20mg morphine.

Morphine sulphate is compatible with all drugs shown in Table 3.2. Diamorphine and oxycodone are also compatible with these drugs, but do show concentration-dependent incompatibility with cyclizine. Diamorphine hydrochloride and cyclizine lactate mixtures are chemically and physically stable in water for injections up to concentrations of 20mg/ml over 24 hours. If the diamorphine concentration exceeds 20mg/ml, crystallization may occur unless the concentration of cyclizine is ≤ 10mg/ml. Similarly, if the concentration of cyclizine exceeds 20mg/ml, crystallization may occur unless the concentration of diamorphine is ≤ 15mg/ml (56). The exact concentrations for oxycodone remain undetermined.

Sedatives

Agitation and delirium in the dying phase are frequently encountered but poorly defined and management can be challenging. Delirium is often unrecognized in patients with advanced cancer and it may be difficult to differentiate between delirium and agitation. Reversible causes should be corrected where possible, although this may not always be practical. Reviewing medication is important, especially as drugs can be implicated in the initiation, aggravation, or perpetuation of delirium. Treatment should include both non-pharmacological and pharmacological measures. The aim of pharmacological treatment should always be to control the agitation or delirium while preserving consciousness. Doses of drugs employed should be titrated to achieve symptom control and while the intention is not to sedate, treatment may at times cause a reduction in the level of consciousness (57). Palliative sedation is defined as 'a medical procedure used to palliate symptoms refractory to standard treatment by intentionally diminishing the conscious level.' (58) This is not practiced in the UK.

Midazolam may be considered the drug of choice for agitation, especially if it is associated with anguish or anxiety. Levomepromazine alone, or in combination with midazolam, should be considered for resistant cases, particularly in patients who are confused, agitated, or experiencing paranoid thoughts. High doses of levomepromazine should not be used without the use of midazolam in patients with brain tumours due to the increased risk of seizures. In patients with delirium, a benzodiazepine may paradoxically exacerbate the condition. The drug treatment of choice for delirium is haloperidol and the dose should be titrated to clinical need (59).

Comfort measures in the last hours or days of life

When it is recognised that the patient's condition has reached the stage where death is imminent there is a need to redefine the goals of the care to be provided. Essentially the patient will be weak and weary; bed-bound and drowsy for long periods; may be disoriented; have an increasing disinterest in food, fluids and in what is happening around them; and possibly finding it difficult to swallow medications. Given this scenario it is essential that any nursing interventions are in the patient's best interest and contribute to a dignified death. In essence all nursing interventions at this stage should be focused on the maintenance of the patient's comfort and safety.

Prior to this stage some elements of care will have simply assisted the caring team to monitor any changes in a patient's condition. Continuing to measure and record vital signs or even to maintain a fluid balance record will in general serve no useful purpose and may even cause discomfort. Regular discussions with the patient and/or family by the nursing team about the patient's comfort will ensure that there is sufficient information to continue an ongoing assessment of care needs and the effectiveness of any interventions that are continued. Any documentation that is maintained should be aimed at ensuring there are no omissions of necessary interventions. The Liverpool Care Pathway for the Dying Patient (LCP) supports this in clinical practice.

Recognition of the dying phase is complex. Therefore, there is a need to assess care that is being delivered and ensure it continues to be in the patient's best interest. Regular reassessment is also important as care needs may change; these goals of care are outlined in the ongoing assessment of the LCP. These goals include micturition, bowel care, mouth care, and skin integrity as well as the monitoring of effective symptom relief.

Mouth care

A dry mouth may be a symptom in the dying patient; its cause is multifactoral including diminished oral intake of fluids, a side effect of medication, and mouth breathing. The current view is that the reduced fluid intake associated with the dying phase is not distressing and that hydration may be detrimental to a patient's comfort (60). The mouth is vital for the maintenance of oral communication and breathing and any problems with the mouth will result in unnecessary additional distress and suffering especially if a dry mouth prevents a patient from being able to speak to their family and friends.

The principles of mouth care for the dying patient are essentially the same as for any other patient and are designed to keep the mouth moist and clean. The major difference is that the patient is unlikely to be able, or want, to take active measures to keep his or her own mouth clean and moist. Thus it is essential for mouth care to be provided for a patient.

Mouth care is an intervention that relatives and carers can be encouraged and enabled to participate in. This may help to give them a sense of being able to do something constructive during the final phase of their loved one's life. If family or carers wish to be involved in their relatives mouth care it is important that they are taught the basic functions of the care and that regular unobtrusive reassessments of the effectiveness of the care being given are made by nurses to ensure that the patient's comfort is maintained.

The type of care necessary will depend on the status of the patient but all dying patients will require assistance to preserve a moist and clean mouth. Assessment is essential and for the dying patient this should focus primarily on how much and what type of assistance the patient requires. Evidence shows that the frequency of mouth care is more important for the maintenance of comfort than either the method of care or the type of fluid used (61). Patients who are either on continuous oxygen therapy, mouth breathing, or unconscious require some type of mouth care at hourly or more frequent intervals if a clean and moist mouth is to be maintained, tailored to individual patient need. Two hourly mouth care will reduce the risk of problems and increase patient comfort (62), but will not usually be sufficient for the maintenance of speech and swallowing. The omission of any type of oral care for between two and four hours will significantly reduce the benefits previously achieved by oral care (63).

For as long as is possible it is preferable that a patient is assisted with his or her own oral hygiene. The provision of regular drinks and giving assistance with tooth brushing can do this effectively. A soft electric toothbrush may be helpful, but there is insufficient evidence to date to support this option. Frequent sips of water, chips of ice to suck, and small chunks of pineapple (in juice not syrup) will all help in keeping a patient's mouth moist and clean. The regular application of Vaseline or a lip salve will also help to maintain moist lips and reduce the risk of cracking and associated discomfort and difficulty in talking.

Current evidence indicates that the use of a soft toothbrush and toothpaste are the best tools for effective mouth care, and especially for removing debris. However, care must be taken to ensure that there is adequate rinsing after the use of toothpaste as it too can cause mouth drying if residue is left on the teeth and in the mouth (64).

The use of mouthwashes may not be appropriate for the dying patient, but where it is possible and a patient is able to tolerate them the type used should be based on patient choice. The efficacy of a mouthwash is achieved from the mechanical action rather than the fluid itself. Recent evidence indicates that normal saline is probably as effective as any other type of solution (62). An alternative for patients who are unable to rinse effectively themselves is to squirt small amount of fluid into the mouth via a syringe, though care must obviously be taken to avoid causing choking.

Saliva substitutes can be used to relieve dryness but most have a short duration of effectiveness and patient preference is for water (65).

Oral care is essential for the maintenance of patient comfort and to enable the dying patient to retain an ability to talk with those closest to him or her. The most effective means of maintaining a moist and clean mouth is by very regular oral care, ie no less than two hourly intervals; and giving the patient the opportunity to have a mouth moisture boost in whichever form the patient prefers, e.g. sips of water, ice chips, or small pieces of pineapple. Saliva replacement gel may be helpful to supplement the natural antibacterial defence system of the mouth, relieves soreness, soothes and protects tissues. The aim is to keep the mouth moist, fresh, and comfortable (Box 3.4).

Micturition difficulties

Urinary dysfunction, either retention or incontinence, has been observed in over 50% of patients during the last 48 hours of life (60). Retention of urine is less likely than incontinence, but either problem may cause additional distress

Box 3.4 Summary points—mouth care

1. Mouth care is vital for the maintenance of oral communication and breathing.

2. Mouth care problems will cause unnecessary additional suffering and distress and may hinder relationships between a patient and those closest to them.

3. Assessment should focus on how much and what type of assistance a patient needs.

4. Frequency of mouth care is more important for the maintenance of comfort than either the method of care or type of fluid used.

5. Relatives and carers can take an active role in the delivery of mouth care.

for the patient and their carers. Urinary output is said to decrease as death approaches (60), the effect of a decrease in urinary output reduces the frequency of micturition and may limit the distress of incontinence and the need for catheterization. Recording how often urine is being passed may assist the team in deciding the ongoing management of any micturition problems and in decisions regarding the use of indwelling urinary catheters.

Urinary retention

The possibility of urinary retention should be considered when a dying patient is restless. Causes of urinary retention include constipation and a full assessment and appropriate treatment plans should be considered according to individualized patient need. For any patient with lower abdominal disease the possibility of cancer causing a direct effect on the bladder must be considered. It is likely that this type of effect will be observed before the patient reaches the dying phase but the possibility should remain a consideration and form part of the ongoing assessment of care needs.

When a patient has urinary retention it is essential to relieve the immediate problem, following a full assessment a urinary catheter may be helpful.

Urinary incontinence

Urinary incontinence may occur in dying patients and may develop as a result of generalized weakness and an inability by the patient to recognize or respond to the sensation of a full bladder. In addition, neurological disturbances or, again, the pressure of a tumour in or on the bladder may result in incontinence.

Some patients may experience frequency of micturition as an effect of bladder irritation from infection or compression from a tumour which may appear as incontinence.

Incontinence can be managed by the use of pads if this is acceptable to the patient and the regular changing of them does not cause additional discomfort.

Catheterization

The question of whether or not to catheterize a dying patient is dependent on a number of factors and the type of micturition problem. Catheterization is used to relieve the problems of retention and incontinence for the dying patient. Careful judgement should be used to ensure that the insertion of a urinary catheter will not cause additional distress and discomfort, especially when it can be anticipated that urinary output will diminish even further as death approaches. Catheterization will of course relieve retention and keep the patient who is incontinent dry, but it should be remembered that catheters may not be comfortable and the action of inserting a catheter, whether it is left *in situ* or not, may cause as much distress as the micturition problem it is aimed at resolving. In such circumstances consideration of the patient's best interest should inform clinical decision making (Box 3.5).

Bowel care

Bowel management during the preceding days and weeks should be sufficiently robust to ensure that the patient is neither constipated nor

---

Box 3.5 Summary points—micturition difficulties

1. Micturition difficulties of any type are distressing for a dying patient although urinary output will diminish as death approaches.

2. Retention of urine is less likely than urinary incontinence, but either problem is common in the last hours or days of life.

3. Retention should be considered when a patient is restless. It may be an effect of either constipation or lower abdominal disease.

4. Catheterization will relieve difficulties of micturition but can be as distressing to patients as either retention or incontinence. Patient preference is paramount.

5. Incontinence can be managed by the use of pads if this is acceptable to the patient.

has diarrhoea. However, as the patient's condition deteriorates bowel activity will diminish and the prospect of constipation, with or without overflow is more likely. Irritation of the bowel by tumour, radiotherapy, or drugs may sometimes result in diarrhoea.

It is inappropriate to consider any bowel intervention unless the patient displays signs or symptoms of a problem. Any problems that do present should be managed to relieve them with the minimum of discomfort for the patient. Constipation can cause agitation and/or urinary retention and thorough assessment of the patient is essential to obtain the correct diagnosis. Similarly, any patient with diarrhoea should be assessed to ensure that it is not constipation with overflow diarrhoea. Gentle rectal and abdominal examination should be sufficient at this stage of the patient's illness.

If a patient is constipated and distressed then a rapid resolution of the problem is essential. Rectal laxatives are often effective because their action is relatively fast and to a certain extent can be controlled and will not be totally dependent on other gut activity. Stimulant suppositories, such as bisacodyl are likely to be the most effective. It is important to remember that any type of rectal intervention may be distressing and should only be used if it is thought to be in the patient's best interest.

The management of diarrhoea is primarily concerned with keeping the patient as clean and comfortable as possible. The administration of additional drugs to relieve diarrhoea will not usually be possible at this stage but could be attempted if the patient is able to tolerate them. Again the gradual slowing of gut activity as the patient's condition deteriorates will cause a lessening, and for many patients cessation, of diarrhoea.

Keeping the patient clean and comfortable in the presence of diarrhoea can be difficult if movement is disturbing. Pads should be positioned in a way that minimizes the amount of disturbance when they are changed. This may require layering of pads so that individual pads can be removed simply by levering the patient rather than having to move or turn the patient frequently, further advice can be sought from a continence advisor. Fragrant oils in the patient's room may help by reducing odour and contribute to the overall comfort (Box 3.6).

Management of skin

Strategies for the prevention of pressure ulcers should have been clearly identified and implemented for individual patients prior to them entering the dying phase. For the dying patient the promotion of dignity and comfort is paramount whilst at the same time there is a need to balance appropriate care with the patient's wishes.

Box 3.6 Summary points—bowel care

1. Following a full assessment it may be appropriate to consider bowel intervention if a dying patient is distressed by either constipation or diarrhoea.

2. Patient agitation can be a sign of constipation.

3. Assessment of patients with diarrhoea should eliminate the possibility of constipation with overflow diarrhoea.

4. Assessment by very gentle rectal examination and abdominal palpation will be sufficient to confirm the diagnosis.

5. Rectal laxatives may be indicated for the essential rapid resolution of constipation in a dying patient.

6. Keeping the patient comfortable and clean is the focus for the management of diarrhoea.

All dying patients are at particular risk of skin breakdown as their deteriorating condition is accompanied by reducing mobility and often cachexia. The degree of risk will to some extent depend on the speed of deterioration but will also be affected by the nature of the disease and the level of existing debility. It is unrealistic to expect healing of pressure ulcers but the use of appropriate pressure relieving aids should help prevent the possibility of the development of further pressure ulcers or exacerbation of existing ones.

Progression into the dying phase should be anticipated and the patient transferred to a high specification pressure relieving mattress/bed as recommended by the NICE guidelines (66). Assessment of the type of bed coverings to be used will be necessary so that skin can be kept as clean and dry as possible.

When a patient is in the last hours or days of life it is essential that careful monitoring of the level of risk continues in a regular and systematic way. This requires a full reassessment of skin integrity at the time it is agreed that the patient is dying and their care is being supported by the LCP. Nurses should continue to use whichever pressure ulcer assessment tool they would normally use for a bed-bound patient, e.g. the Waterlow Score or the Braden Score to support clinical judgement. Whichever tool is used, it is likely that a dying patient will fall into the high or very high risk category and will therefore need the use of pressure relieving aids to promote comfort. (Box 3.7).

When a diagnosis of dying is made and the LCP is used to support care delivery for a patient, it does not diminish the amount of nursing care a patient requires. On the contrary for many patients the amount of direct nursing care

Box 3.7 Summary points—pressure area care/mobility

1 All dying patients will be at a high risk of skin breakdown.

2. Care should focus on the prevention of further deterioration of existing pressure ulcers and the development of new ones.

3. Generally patients will need a high specification pressure relieving mattress/bed as recommended by the NICE guidelines (66).

4. Regular reassessment of skin integrity is supported by the LCP.

will increase during the dying phase. The family and caregivers also need regular support and assistance including clear communication and appropriate information. Care of the dying is urgent care with one opportunity to ensure a dignified death for the patient and the opportunity for a positive lasting memory for those who live on after a loved one has died.

References

1 A controlled trial to improve care for seriously ill hospitalized patients. The study to understand prognoses and preferences for outcomes and risks of treatments (SUPPORT). The SUPPORT Principal Investigators. *JAMA* 1995;**274**:1591–8.

2 Ellershaw J, Foster A, Murphy D, et al. Developing an integrated care pathway for the dying patient. *Eur J Palliat Care* 1997;**4**:203–7.

3 Overill S. A practical guide to integrated pathways. *J Integrated Care* 1998;**2**:93–8.

4 Ellershaw J, Ward C. Care of the dying patient: the last hours or days of life. *BMJ* 2003;**326**:30–4.

5 Finucane TE. How gravely ill becomes dying: a key to end-of-life care. *JAMA* 1999;**282**:1670–2.

6 Lichter I, Hunt E. The last 48 hours of life. *J Palliat Care* 1990;**6**:7–15.

7 Turner K, Chye R, Aggarwal G, et al. Dignity in dying: a preliminary study of patients in the last three days of life. *J Palliat Care* 1996;**12**:7–13.

8 Nauck F, Klachik E, Ostgathe C. Symptom control during the last three days of life. *Eur J Palliat Care* 2001;**10**:81–4.

9 Ellershaw J. Care of the dying: what a difference an LCP makes! *Palliat Med* 2007;**21**:365–8.

10 Mullick A, Beynon T, Colvin M, et al. Liverpool care pathway carers survey. *Palliat Med* 2009;**23**:571–2.

11 Ellershaw J, Smith C, Overill S, et al. Care of the dying: setting standards for symptom control in the last 48 hours of life. *J Pain Symptom Manage* 2001;**21**:12–17.

12 Veerbeek L, van Zuylen L, Swart SJ, et al. The effect of the Liverpool Care Pathway for the dying: a multi-centre study. *Palliat Med* 2008;**22**:145–51.

13 Bookbinder M, Blank AE, Arney E, et al. Improving end-of-life care: development and pilot-test of a clinical pathway. *J Pain Symptom Manage* 2005;**29**:529–43.

14 Jarabek BR, Jama AA, Cha SS, et al. Use of a palliative care order set to improve resident comfort with symptom management in palliative care. *Palliat Med* 2008;**22**:343–9.

15 Centeno C, Sanz A, Bruera E. Delirium in advanced cancer patients. *Palliat Med* 2004;**18**:184–94

16 Lawlor PG, Gagnon B, Mancini IL, et al. Occurrence, causes, and outcome of delirium in patients with advanced cancer: a prospective study. *Arch Intern Med* 2000;**160**:786–94.

17 Breitbart W, Strout D. Delirium in the terminally ill. *Clin Geriatr Med* 2000; **16**:357–72.

18 Goncalves JF, Alvarenga M, Silva A. The last forty-eight hours of life in a Portuguese palliative care unit: does it differ from elsewhere? *J Palliat Med* 2003;**6**:895–900.

19 Fainsinger R, Miller MJ, Bruera E, et al. Symptom control during the last week of life on a palliative care unit. *J Palliat Care* 1991;**7**:5–11.

20 Grond S, Zech D, Schug SA, et al. Validation of World Health Organization guidelines for cancer pain relief during the last days and hours of life. *J Pain Symptom Manage* 1991;**6**:411–22.

21 Conill C, Verger E, Henriquez I, et al. Symptom prevalence in the last week of life. *J Pain Symptom Manage* 1997;**14**:328–31.

22 Greaves J, Glare P, Kristjanson LJ, et al. Undertreatment of nausea and other symptoms in hospitalized cancer patients. *Support Care Cancer* 2009;**17**:461–4.

23 Twycross RG, Lack SA. *Symptom control in far advanced cancer: pain relief*. Pitman, London, 1983.

24 Virik K, Glare P. Pain management in palliative care. Reviewing the issues. *Aust Fam Physician* 2000;**29**:1027–33.

25 Lickiss JN. Approaching cancer pain relief. *Eur J Pain* 2001;**5** Suppl A:5–14.

26 Twycross RG, Lack SA. *Therapeutics in terminal cancer*. Churchill Livingstone, Edinburgh,1990.

27 Bruera E, Franco JJ, Maltoni M, et al. Changing pattern of agitated impaired mental status in patients with advanced cancer: association with cognitive monitoring, hydration, and opioid rotation. *J Pain Symptom Manage* 1995;**10**:287–91.

28 Eisele JH Jr, Grigsby EJ, Dea G. Clonazepam treatment of myoclonic contractions associated with high-dose opioids: case report. *Pain* 1992;**49**:231–2.

29 Bruera E, Sala R, Rico MA, et al. Effects of parenteral hydration in terminally ill cancer patients: a preliminary study. *J Clin Oncol* 2005;**23**:2366–71.

30 Clary PL, Lawson P. Pharmacologic pearls for end-of-life care. *Am Fam Physician* 2009;**79**:1059–65.

31 Furst CJ, Doyle D. The terminal phase, in Doyle D, Hanks G, Cherny N, et al. (eds): *Oxford textbook of palliative medicine*. Oxford University Press, Oxford 2004, 1119–33.

32 Davies AN, Dickman A, Reid C, Stevens AM, Zeppetella G. The management of cancer-related breakthrough pain: Recommendations of a task group of the Science Committee of the Association for Palliative Medicine of Great Britain and Ireland. *Eur J Pain*. 2009;**13**(4):331–8.

33 Portenoy RK, Sibirceva U, Smout R, et al. Opioid use and survival at the end of life: a survey of a hospice population. *J Pain Symptom Manage* 2006;**32**:532–40.

34 Portenoy RK, Thomas J, Moehl Boatwright ML, et al. Subcutaneous methylnaltrexone for the treatment of opioid-induced constipation in patients with advanced illness: a double-blind, randomized, parallel group, dose-ranging study. *J Pain Symptom Manage* 2008;**35**:458–68.

35 Agar M, Currow D, Plummer J, et al. Changes in anticholinergic load from regular prescribed medications in palliative care as death approaches. *Palliat Med* 2009; **23**:257–65.

36 Macleod AD. The management of delirum in hospice practice. *Eur J Palliat Care* 1997;**4**:116–20.

37 Breitbart W, Alici Y. Agitation and delirium at the end of life: 'We couldn't manage him'. *JAMA* 2008;**300**:2898–910, E1.

38 Spiller JA, Keen JC. Hypoactive delirium: assessing the extent of the problem for inpatient specialist palliative care. *Palliat Med* 2006;**20**:17–23.

39 Ventafridda V, Ripamonti C, De Conno F, et al. Symptom prevalence and control during cancer patients' last days of life. *J Palliat Care* 1990;**6**:7–11.

40 Fainsinger RL, De Moissac D, Mancini I, et al. Sedation for delirium and other symptoms in terminally ill patients in Edmonton. *J Palliat Care* 2000;**16**:5–10.

41 Rietjens JA, van Zuylen L, van Veluw H, et al. Palliative sedation in a specialized unit for acute palliative care in a cancer hospital: comparing patients dying with and without palliative sedation. *J Pain Symptom Manage* 2008;**36**:228–34.

42 Connor SR, Pyenson B, Fitch K, et al. Comparing hospice and nonhospice patient survival among patients who die within a three-year window. *J Pain Symptom Manage* 2007;**33**:238–46.

43 McIver B, Walsh D, Nelson K, The use of chlorpromazine for symptom control in dying cancer patients. *J Pain Symptom Manage* 1994;**9**:341–5.

44 Boettger S, Breitbart W. Atypical antipsychotics in the management of delirium: a review of the empirical literature. *Palliat Support Care* 2005;**3**:227–37.

45 de Graeff A, Dean M. Palliative sedation therapy in the last weeks of life: a literature review and recommendations for standards. *J Palliat Med* 2007;**10**:67–85.

46 Bennett MI. Death rattle: An audit of hyoscine (scopolamine) use and review of management. *J Pain Symptom Manage* 1996;**12**:229–33.

47 Ellershaw JE, Sutcliffe JM, Saunders CM. Dehydration and the dying patient. *J Pain Symptom Manage* 1995;**10**:192–97.

48 Wildiers H, Dhaenekint C, Demeulenaere P et al. Atropine, hyoscine butylbromide, or scopolamine are equally effective for the treatment of death rattle in terminal care. *J Pain Symptom Manage.* 2009;**38**(1):124–33.

49 Hugel H, Ellershaw J, Gambles M. Respiratory tract secretions in the dying patient: a comparison between glycopyrronium and hyoscine hydrobromide. *J Palliat Med* 2006;**9**(2):279–84.

50 Wee B, Hillier R. Interventions for noisy breathing in patients near to death. *Cochrane Database of Syst Rev.* 2008; 1: CD005177. DOI: 10.1002/14651858.CD005177.pub2.

51 Hughes A, Wilcock A, Corcoran R, Lucas V, King A. Audit of three antimuscarinic drugs for managing retained secretions. *Palliat Med* 2000;**14**:221–22.

52 Doyle J, Walker P, Bruera E. Nebulized scopolamine. *J Pain Symptom Manage.* 2000;**19**:327–28.

53 Cranston JM, Crockett A, Currow D. Oxygen therapy for dyspnoea in adults. *Cochrane Database of Systematic Reviews* 2008; 3: CD004769. DOI: 10.1002/14651858.CD004769.pub2.

54 Viola R, Kiteley C, Lloyd NS et al. The management of dyspnea in cancer patients: a systematic review. *Support Care Cancer* 2008;**16**:329–37.

55 O'Doherty CA, Hall EJ, Schofield L, Zeppetella G. Drugs and syringe drivers: a survey of adult specialist palliative care practice in the United Kingdom and Eire. *Palliat Med* 2001;**15**:149–54.

56 Dickman A, Schneider J, Varga J. *The Syringe Driver: Continuous Subcutaneous Infusions in Palliative Care.* Second Ed Oxford University Press. Oxford. 2005.

57 De Graeff A, Dean M. Palliative Sedation Therapy in the Last Weeks of Life: A Literature Review and Recommendations for Standards. *J Palliat Med* 2007;**10**:67–85.

58 Morita T, Tsunoda J, Inoue S, Chihara S. Do hospice clinicians sedate patients intending to hasten death? *J Palliat Care* 1999;**15**(3): 20–23.

59 Gagnon PR. Treatment of delirium in supportive and palliative care. Curr Opin *Support Palliat Care* 2008;**2**(1):60–6.

60 Fürst and Doyle, D. (2005). In *Oxford textbook of palliative medicine* (ed. D. Doyle, G. Hanks, N. Cherny and K. Calman, Chapter 18. Oxford Medical Publications, Oxford.

61 Duxbury, A., Thakker, N., and Wastell,D. A double-blind crossover trial of a mucin containing artificial saliva. *Br. Dent. J* 1989;**166**;115–20.

62 Homes, S. Nursing management of oral care in older patients. *Nurs. Times*, 1996;**92**; 37–8.

63 Howarth, H. Mouth care procedures for the very ill. *Nurs. Times*, 1997;**93**;345–55.

64 Holmes,S. The oral complications of specific anticancer therapy. *International Journal of Nursing*, 1991;**28**,(4); 173–7.

65 Miller, M. and Kearney, N. Oral care for patients with cancer: A review of the literature. *Cancer Nurs.* 2001;**24**:241–4.

66 NICE (2005). *The prevention and treatment of pressure ulcers. Guideline 29*, National Institute for Health and Clinical Excellence www.nice.org/CG029.

Chapter 4

Ethical issues in care of the dying

Andrew Thorns and Eve Garrard

What is the moral justification for the Liverpool Care Pathway?

The Liverpool Care Pathway for the Dying Patient (LCP) aims to provide the most effective clinical care to patients in the last hours or days of life. It does not remove clinical judgement about which action provides overall benefit for the patient nor does it influence outcomes, provided it is used appropriately. Therefore the LCP provides a benefit to patients with no correlative harm; hence professionals looking after patients at the end of life have a responsibility to make appropriate use of this procedure.

How can the Liverpool Care Pathway for the Dying Patient influence ethical decision making?

The aim of care pathways is to promote the principle of high quality care, and this applies to ethical issues just as much as to other aspects of patient and family care.

Health care professionals frequently find themselves trying to make difficult ethical decisions at the end of a patient's life. The right course of action may not be clear, leaving professionals anxious that morally or legally they are acting inappropriately. Common examples might include decisions about withholding or withdrawing treatments, or about the use of sedation or analgesia for symptom control. Failure to address such issues adequately can interfere with good patient care if it leads to the patient continuing with burdensome treatments or being denied the relief of discomfort. Therefore, it is important to monitor ethical decisions, show how they are justified, and continuously aim to improve them.

The patient, relatives, and friends may also be concerned about these ethical issues as a result of coverage by the media. They will want both reassurance that the health care team is acting correctly and also the opportunity for discussion. In order to meet these needs health care professionals have to be confident of their own position. The LCP makes it possible to incorporate available evidence and national or regional policies into decision making at the end of life, and thereby to promote good practice. When difficult decisions are required the health care professional can then feel reassured both in moral as well as in legal terms.

Advice contained in the LCP can only be presented in general terms. Central to care of the dying is the recognition that the decision making process has to be tailored to the individual. The information contained in this chapter, when used alongside the LCP, can facilitate this process, but must be supplemented by effective multidisciplinary team working and sensitive communication skills. The correct moral action may at times be clear, but communicating such decisions in highly emotive situations is often a challenging task. There is little point in arriving at the correct moral decision if the necessary skills are not available to communicate this to the people involved.

An ethical framework

What is the best approach to ethical decision making?

A common approach to ethical decision making is the 'Four Principles' approach presented by Beauchamp and Childress (1). They suggest that there are four moral principles which govern the field of health care ethics, namely the principles of:

- Respect for autonomy
- Beneficence: the duty to provide benefit
- Non-maleficence: the duty not to harm
- Distributive justice: the fair use and distribution of resources

Although there is some debate about whether these principles are sufficient to cover the whole of health care ethics, many health care ethicists think that they do cover a great deal of it, and at the very least provide a good starting point. By considering the role and importance of each of these principles in a given situation we can hope to come to a reasonable moral decision about how to act.

Respect for autonomy

The principle of respect for autonomy recognizes the individual's right to decide upon their own destiny and to be in charge of decisions relating to themselves. In order to act autonomously an individual needs to be fully informed, competent to retain and process that information in deciding on the best course of action, and free from manipulative or coercive pressures. We cannot, therefore, respect our patient's autonomy simply by offering them a choice. We need also to ensure that they have adequate information and are not inappropriately pressured by others to choose one way rather than another.

The principle of respect for autonomy also requires that the autonomy of other members of society should be respected. There may be times when a patient's autonomous decision has to be rejected because of its effect on others. In fact, patients entering onto the LCP are unlikely to be competent to act in an autonomous manner. However it does not follow that the principle of respect for autonomy is inapplicable in their case, a point which will be discussed in more detail later.

Beneficence and non-maleficence

Beneficence is the duty to act in a way that provides benefit to others, and non-maleficence is the duty not to harm. Benefits incorporate not only the clinical success of an intervention, but also emotional and other factors relevant to the patient's welfare (3). These would appear to be obvious principles to follow, both being part of our common sense understanding of morality. It is important, however, to remember that neither is absolute. A certain degree of harm may be necessary to provide a benefit, or the opportunity to benefit a patient may be outweighed by a duty to respect one of the other principles. A patient, for example, may decline a potentially life-saving procedure for their own individual reasons, going against what the health care professional may perceive as a benefit; and here respect for patient autonomy may outweigh the demands of the principle of beneficence.

Perhaps the most difficult consideration is how to determine or measure what constitutes a benefit or harm to an individual. This will vary from one person to another and generally is an assessment that is best left to the patient. However in the last few days of life the patient is unlikely to be able to help with such decisions. The health care professional, in consultation with those close to the patient, is then left working out how to benefit or avoid harming the patient, and also how that should be balanced against other relevant considerations.

Justice

The principle of justice refers to distributive justice: the fair use and distribution of resources. (It does not refer to criminal justice in the health care context). At first sight, it appears to be intuitively right that resources should be divided equally between all members of society. However, criteria other than equality are also important—for example, the level of need in a particular patient, or the likelihood that the health care intervention will be successful. Ensuring fair distribution seems particularly important in health care where resources are limited and the boundaries of health needs are vague. Respecting the principle of justice can result in difficult decisions.

At the end of life the right to scarce resources may seem to be less important as death is inevitable and close. Certainly expensive interventions with negligible chance of benefit should be discontinued, but some resources are usefully invested in this group. Not only do we have a moral obligation to meet the needs of symptom control and nursing care, we must also consider the more widespread benefit during the bereavement phase to those close to the patient. A peaceful death with well-informed and supported relatives is likely to be emotionally less upsetting for all concerned, possibly with less use of services in bereavement.

The term 'resources' need not only refer to financial resources; professional time is another important resource that needs to be divided equitably. Health care professionals commonly find themselves divided between a number of responsibilities and have to decide where their time is best spent. A nurse who has two patients requiring his or her help at the same time has to decide which patient to go to first. How should such decisions be made? Usually a consideration of the degree of benefit would be foremost for the health care professional in such a situation. It is easy to see how the dying patient might take second place to the patient who is likely to be cured. It is equally easy to see the stress that can result from making such decisions.

Withholding and withdrawing interventions and treatments at the end of life

What is an effective approach when making decisions about withholding and withdrawing treatment?

Commonly ethical dilemmas approaching the end of life revolve around decisions to withhold or withdraw interventions or treatment (2). When the patient and doctor agree that there is no benefit to carrying on or starting a new intervention the right action is clear, though skill is required on the doctor's part to manage these discussions sensitively.

Professionals have a responsibility to develop a just approach to withholding and withdrawing treatments and interventions at the end of life (Fig.4.1)(3).

One such approach is suggested in Box 4.1 demonstrating the different layers which need to be considered in arriving at the best action. The elements of each layer will be considered in relation to common clinical dilemmas.

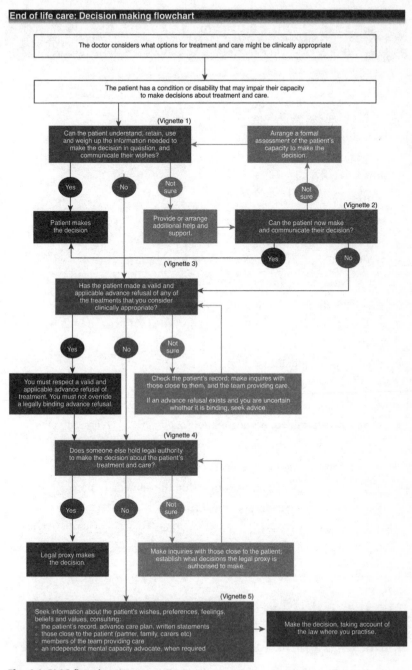

Fig. 4.1 GMC flowchart.
See GMC website for full document (3). Reproduced with the permission of the
General Medical Council

Box 4.1 The layered approach to decisions to withhold or withdraw an intervention or treatment

Layer 1: The framework or facts—what we are bound by?

- The law
- Professional guidance
- Evidence base
- Resources available

Layer 2: The patient

- Their capacity
- Their beliefs and preferences
- Prognosis/outlook/likely changes in condition
- Other nominated decision makers where appropriate

Layer 3: Formulating the ethical problem

- Ensure the correct question(s) is being asked
- Ensure we are not being inappropriately influenced by our own perspective

Layer 4: Establishing the options

- What are the potential moral justifications?
- What are the practical solutions?
- What communication/negotiation/explanation is required?

Layer 5: Communicating and coordinating

- Communicating the options to those involved
- Coordinating and putting into action the decision making
- Reviewing the decision on a regular basis

This encompasses the decision making pathway produced by the GMC in their guidance *Treatment and care towards the end of life: Good practice in decision making* (4) which is shown in Figure 4.1.

If there is a decision between a treatment that will prolong life and one that will only promote comfort, should the right action always be one that extends life?

The clinical team must start from a presumption in favour of prolonging life and must not be motivated by a desire to shorten life if considering withdrawing or withholding a treatment.

There is not a responsibility to always preserve life (4). A treatment aimed at comfort instead of prolonging life is indicated when:

◆ This is the autonomous decision of the patient (see the case of Ms B (5))

◆ The harms or side effects of the life-prolonging treatment outweigh any benefit

◆ The quality of life is so poor that the patient and the professionals agree not to start the life-prolonging treatment.

However it is clear that if there is any doubt the clinical team should opt to prolong life (4,6).

Cardiopulmonary resuscitation (CPR)

What should be the approach when CPR is thought to offer no chance of success?

For patients on the LCP, the evidence is clear that attempting CPR is rarely, if ever, a life-saving procedure (7,8). It is instead an unnecessary and disturbing intervention. Even in the exceptional cases where it does re-establish some cardiac function, this will only result in a short period of significantly impaired quality life. In these cases CPR is to be rejected on grounds of futility.

This should be clearly distinguished from other circumstances when a decision is based on the patient's quality of life where there is a reasonable chance of surviving CPR.

Decisions relating to CPR have attracted a great deal of public attention. Many people have expressed fears about the withholding of a potentially life-saving procedure without prior discussion with the patient or relative. Such fears suggest that there is widespread misunderstanding of the nature and likely success of CPR procedures. This misperception may be perpetuated by popular television dramas portraying unrealistic success rates from CPR (9,10).

The decision about whether attempts at CPR will be successful is a clinical one and the final responsibility for this assessment lies with the doctor in charge of the patient's care.

If 'not for CPR' is to be recorded in the notes, is it necessary to discuss this with the patient and the family?

Discussion is important regarding future management, but this needs to be tailored to individual requirements and need not specifically include CPR. However assumptions should not be made about a patient's preferences. Sensitive exploration of how willing they might be to know about a 'do not attempt cardiopulmonary resuscitation' (DNACPR) decision should be undertaken (4). While some patients may want to be told, others may find discussion about interventions that would not be clinically appropriate burdensome and of little or no value. You should not withhold information simply because conveying it is difficult or uncomfortable for you or the healthcare team. CPR is just one end of life issue out of many. When it is likely to be futile, discussion of CPR as a separate consideration may only reinforce the misperception of it as having life-saving properties.

Some patients and families will be satisfied with more general discussions of the future, others will want more detailed discussions. To include CPR in these more detailed discussions would be appropriate.

How is the discussion with the patient, family, or carer best approached?

Discussing the clinical situation regularly with patients and, with permission, families and carers is fundamental to good care. Rather than focus on specific issues such as CPR however, this discussion should focus on the fact that the patient is now dying. It should centre on their understanding of the patient's current condition, that there are no more active treatment options, so the focus will now be on comfort and maintaining dignity. Practical issues are also important, such as the need to arrange time off from work, or to contact members of the family or friends. The emphasis should be on what is for the patient's overall benefit rather than interventions that will not offer any benefit. In the course of such discussion there would be little benefit in specifically initiating a discussion of attempted CPR, when it is accepted that the patient is dying. An exception to this approach would be for patients dying at home. In order to prevent unnecessary calls to the emergency services, the fact that CPR and other resuscitation techniques should not be started as they offer no benefit should be made clear.

These discussions should always be recorded in the patient record and a DNACPR form completed. Apart from the obvious legal reasons for this it also informs other members of the team of the situation.

What if families or friends ask about CPR?

Families may wish to raise the issue of CPR specifically. It is useful to begin such discussion by gaining an understanding of their perceptions of CPR and what they hope it would achieve. The harm caused by CPR in terms of lack of dignity and possible pain and discomfort to the patient with no resulting life prolongation are the key issues to discuss. The moral justification of not attempting CPR with patients on the LCP rests on these issues.

Should families or friends be asked to make CPR decisions?

Asking families or friends to make decisions about attempting futile CPR can be harmful. Without the clinical knowledge families may feel they have denied the patient a life-saving procedure, perhaps causing their death. This misperception can be a source of great anxiety and may make the bereavement process more difficult.

Are guidelines available to help decision making on CPR?

The fears raised by the public have resulted in a number of organizations producing guidelines which aim to allay these fears and at the same time promote good practice amongst clinicians. As a result all health care organizations should have a written policy relating to decisions about CPR. Guidance from the Association for Palliative Medicine and the National Council for Hospice and Palliative Care Services states that discussion of futile CPR with all patients is not indicated (11). The British Medical Association, the Resuscitation Council (UK), and the Royal College of Nursing produced *Decisions relating to cardiopulmonary resuscitation* (12) in 2007. The General Medical Council published their guidance in May 2010 (4).

What are the ethical implications of implantable cardiac defibrillators (ICDs)?

ICDs will offer no benefit to patients who are dying and who meet the criteria to be placed on the LCP. The risk of them delivering a shock to the patient in the dying phase is prevented by de-activating them in advance. This area of practice has been covered in more detail by the British Heart Foundation document *Implantable cardioverter defibrillators in patients who are reaching the end of life* (13).

Issues of hydration and nutrition

If the patient is no longer taking fluids by mouth, is it ethical not to hydrate them with intravenous or subcutaneous fluids?

The provision of hydration is an essential part of human flourishing. Families and professionals are understandably concerned with the thought of withdrawing clinically assisted hydration including in the last days or hours of life.

When hydration becomes clinically assisted it is classed as a treatment rather than basic care. Therefore, when it ceases to offer any benefit, it can legitimately be withdrawn (4,6). However, a recent systematic review has highlighted the lack of robust evidence to support decision making in this area (14). Traditional thinking in palliative care has held that the harms from providing clinically assisted hydration usually outweigh any benefits.

The key issue is to distinguish a patient who is dying from their disease from one who is dying because they are unable to maintain their hydration. If the patient is not in the dying phase, then clinically assisted hydration may well be indicated. A patient who is confused, with an infection or a metabolic disturbance such as hypercalcaemia, may gain significant benefit from rehydration. Similarly a patient with a physical obstruction, such as carcinoma of the oesophagus, may need clinically assisted hydration (or nutrition) until the obstruction can be resolved. Patients commencing the LCP should have had such conditions excluded.

In the last few days or hours of life, the moral basis for withdrawing or withholding clinically assisted hydration rests on the benefits and harms to the patient. Patients are often only able to take sips of fluid and as they approach death they are unlikely to be taking anything by mouth. This appears to be a natural process and experience in palliative care suggests that the majority of patients die quite peacefully and comfortably without the use of clinically assisted hydration. It is likely that symptoms associated with a dry mouth are caused more by medication and mouth breathing than by lack of fluid. Appropriate mouth care would be the most effective way to counter this symptom.

There are a number of potential risks or harms from clinically assisted hydration including excess respiratory secretions, oedema, and site problems from the intravenous or subcutaneous infusions. Equipment may interfere with contact between the patient and families at an emotionally sensitive time.

In this case it is not that the patient is dying from a lack of hydration, but that they are dying and so do not require it (15,16). Therefore, it is usually in the patient's overall benefit not to receive clinically assisted hydration and so withholding it is morally justified.

The professional will need to explore and understand the ideas, concerns, and expectations of the patient and family. Usually a discussion of the lack of benefit of clinically assisted hydration leaves families in favour of the decision. However, if strong concerns remain, a trial of clinically assisted hydration may reassure them that such an intervention will not benefit their relative. Regular review of the situation is required whichever decision is made.

If the benefits and burdens are finely balanced, the patient's wishes will usually be determinative.

If the patient already has clinically assisted hydration in place, is it ethical to discontinue it when they are placed on the LCP?

To discontinue clinically assisted hydration in this situation is entirely justifiable. The answer to the previous question addresses how clinically assisted hydration offers little or no benefit to the patient but does involve potential harms, and therefore why it is usual practice not to commence this intervention.

Intuitively it seems that to take something away is harder to justify than not commencing the intervention in the first place. However, if we consider how the four principles apply to this situation the arguments remain the same as in the previous question. The right action here remains a balance of the benefits against harms. The fact that clinically assisted hydration is already being provided does not influence this. The key aspect is the intention of the health care professional. In withdrawing clinically assisted hydration the health care professional intends to improve the overall comfort of the patient and to try to prevent any harm. This is the same intention as the health care professional who decides not to start hydration.

If a patient has been diagnosed as being in a persistent vegetative state the courts in England, Wales, and Northern Ireland currently require that you approach them for a ruling before withdrawing clinically assisted nutrition and hydration (CANH).

How does the approach to clinically assisted nutrition differ to this?

The same considerations apply to nutrition as do to hydration. Whilst again there is little robust evidence to support decisions in this area (15,17), professionals need to ask whether the patient is one who is dying from their disease rather than from a lack of nutrition. If clinically assisted nutrition offers no benefit (it is futile) then it can be withheld or withdrawn for the same reasons as hydration.

Issues of ventilation

What is the ethical approach to a patient's request to withdraw ventilation?

The framework can be applied in the same way as for CPR and hydration and nutrition. One widely-known example of this is the case of Ms B, a patient with capacity who wished to have her ventilation stopped despite knowing that this would result in her death. The court upheld her request, taking the view that the responsibility to respect this autonomous decision outweighed the harm from stopping treatment (5).

In such cases there will be a need for effective symptom control whilst the ventilation is withdrawn.

What is the ethical approach to withdrawing ventilation when the patient doesn't want to?

When the ventilation is thought to be offering no benefit and yet the patient wants to continue with it, this creates an ethically challenging situation.

Applying the four principles approach will generally show that as a matter of respecting the patient's autonomy the ventilation should be continued. The principle of distributive justice would suggest stopping ventilation as it is an unnecessary use of resources. The professionals are likely to feel that the harms of the treatment outweigh any benefit. But the patient's perspective of these harms and benefits may be different, and in this case that is likely to outweigh other considerations. This is a good example of where there is a need for effective communication skills and symptom control to manage such dilemmas.

How does the approach to withdrawing or withholding dialysis compare to ventilation?

The same principles and approach apply to the withdrawal or withholding of dialysis as to ventilation.

Shortening and ending life: the doctrine of double effect and assisted dying

What is the difference between euthanasia, assisted suicide, and assisted dying?

Euthanasia is defined as the intentional bringing about of the death of a patient, either by killing him or by allowing him to die, for the patient's own sake.

Physician-assisted suicide (PAS) is similar except that the patient administers the lethal dose themselves. Assisted dying is a term that incorporates both. These practices remain illegal in the UK, although there is greater acceptance of this practice in some other countries.

If a patient is dying and is given medication to relieve symptoms e.g. subcutaneous morphine for pain, and then dies a few minutes later, is this euthanasia?

Opioids, such as morphine, provide effective relief for the frequently distressing symptoms of pain and dyspnoea as the end of life approaches. However there is a frequent misconception amongst professionals that if they increase the doses of these drugs or give an extra dose, the life of the patient may be shortened—a belief also often shared by patients and their families. If this were indeed the case, the doctrine of double effect (DDE), if legitimate, would provide moral justification for such a consequence, but this raises a concern that it may protect dangerous practice.

What the DDE says is that an action (such as giving a dose of opioid) where the professional foresees it may shorten life but does not aim at this outcome, is morally justified provided the intention is to benefit the patient and not to shorten their life. Because the professional isn't aiming at the death of the patient, this cannot count as a case of euthanasia.

In the classic version of a case to which the DDE applies, the situation is that a patient is in pain. A dose of opioid is given to relieve that pain but at the same time the health care professional believes that this may shorten life. But this traditional argument has come under increasing challenge (Box 4.2) (18–20). The main reason for this challenge is the fact that opioids used in line with best practice do not risk shortening life. With effective specialist palliative care it is rare that doses need to be increased to such levels that the patient's life may be put at risk.

Any professional who feels that they may be shortening a patient's life by the use of opioids or sedatives should contact specialist palliative care services for advice.

Therefore the health care professional in this situation is not performing euthanasia as it is unlikely their action caused or hastened the death, and in any case their intention is only to relieve symptoms. Nonetheless health care professionals are often left with a feeling that it was their action in giving or prescribing the last injection that caused the death. This is a feeling that may be uncomfortable. However, we know that symptoms worsen as death approaches, and so increased use of symptomatic treatments is therefore likely to be necessary. Death might well have occurred at that time even without intervention.

Is the use of sedative drugs justified in the same way?

Morally and legally the use of sedative medication to achieve symptom control is justified in the same manner (Box 4.3). The use of opioids is quite specific for pain or dyspnoea. The potential role for sedative drugs in managing symptoms or psychological issues that can't be resolved in other ways is much broader. Estimates vary but sedation results from the relief of unendurable symptoms in about 15–36% of patients in some palliative care units (21). This may appear ethically more concerning as the treatment is less specific, more open to abuse, and seems intuitively more difficult to justify. However, the principles previously discussed apply similarly here. An agitated, anxious, confused, or breathless dying patient causes distress not only to themselves but to all those watching. At times the use of medication which results in sedation may be the only way to offer relief and in these circumstances is considered essential for effective symptom control at the end of life. A number of studies have suggested that survival is not affected when sedative drugs are used in line with accepted practice (20).

Box 4.2 Association for Palliative Medicine position statement on the doctrine of double effect in end of life care

1. The Association for Palliative Medicine (APM) is an organization of over 1000 specialist palliative care doctors working in hospices, hospitals, and the community.

2. The Double Effect (sometimes called a rule, principle, or doctrine) states that 'The risk of a potential, known (foreseen), unintended consequence or side effect of treatment is justified only if all the following criteria are met:
   - The intended effect is good in itself
   - The clinician's intention is solely to produce the good effect
   - The intervention is proportionate to the situation
   - The good effect is not achieved through the bad effect'.

3. There is a misconception that morphine related drugs and sedative drugs bring about death more quickly and that doctors both know this and in some way condone their use with reference to the double effect.

4. The APM refutes this claim: it knows of no credible research evidence to suggest that a patient's life is shortened either by opioids or sedatives when used in line with accepted palliative care practice.

5. The APM believes that the double effect is unnecessary to justify the use of dosing regimes necessary to manage pain or distress in all but the most exceptional circumstances.

6. Professionals who are concerned they are shortening life by the use of these medications should contact their local specialist palliative care services.

When will a professional involved in end of life care be at risk of prosecution for assisting suicide?

Assisting suicide remains a criminal offence in the United Kingdom. However the Director for Public Prosecutions has issued guidance for when prosecutions are not thought to be in the public's best interest (22). Professionals involved in patient care are still advised not to give advice or resources that might aid a suicide (23).

Box 4.3 Association for Palliative Medicine position on the use of sedation at the end of life

1. The Association for Palliative Medicine is an organization of over 1000 specialist palliative care doctors working in hospices, hospitals and the community.

2. All medication used in palliative care, including sedative medication, is aimed at the relief of specific symptoms.

3. Medication which is sedating in its effect should only be used if the symptom cannot be relieved with more specific interventions.

4. Rarely, patients may experience distress when symptoms cannot be controlled even after exhaustive attempts with specific interventions. In these circumstances some patients may require sedating medication to diminish awareness of their suffering.

5. If medication is sedating in its effect, the dose should be monitored in order to ensure that it is the minimum required to relieve the patient's distress. Medication used in this way does not shorten life.

6. Sedation in palliative care is thus sedation while the patient dies and is not sedating the patient to death.

7. Morphine and related drugs are vital painkillers but are wholly unsuitable for use as sedation.

Issues relating to capacity and decision making

When a patient lacks capacity, what does the law require of health professionals in making decisions for them?

The Mental Capacity Act (2005) in England and Wales and the Adults with Incapacity Act (2000) in Scotland detail the steps required by professionals in assessing capacity and making decisions for patients who are shown to lack capacity for that decision. For this section we shall refer to the MCA (2005) and its associated guidance (24). This would need to be confirmed in areas outside England and Wales.

How should the capacity of the patient be assessed?

The assessment of capacity is specific to the decision being made. The MCA (2005) details the steps required of professionals in making this assessment (Box 4.4).

Box 4.4 Requirements to demonstrate a lack of capacity for decision making

The MCA requirements to demonstrate a lack of capacity are:

◆ Is there an impairment of, or disturbance in, the functioning of the person's mind or brain?

◆ Is the impairment or disturbance sufficient to cause the person to be unable to make that particular decision at the relevant time?

When it is suspected that a person has a loss of capacity because of impaired functioning of the mind or brain, he/she must also be unable to do at least one of the following:

◆ understand the information about the proposed intervention (which must be imparted in a manner which can realistically be understood, such as via an interpreter)

◆ retain that information (even if only for a short period)

◆ use or weigh that information

◆ communicate the decision (by any means).

This assessment is decision-specific and time-specific (24).

If the multidisciplinary team decide that a patient is in the dying phase, but the relatives want all active treatment to be continued, how should the views of the relatives influence the decision making of the multidisciplinary team?

The ultimate responsibility for treatment decisions lies with the patient and the doctor in charge of their care. If there is disagreement between the doctor and the patient or those close to the patient, the GMC suggests the steps described in Box 4.5 should be taken. Doctors cannot treat patients with capacity against their will, but neither can they be forced to provide a treatment that has no benefit to the patient. The approach to this situation starts with an assessment of the patient's capacity for the decision in question. It is the responsibility of the professional to demonstrate that a patient lacks capacity, however the majority of patients supported by the LCP are likely to be only semi-conscious and therefore unable to make decisions for themselves.

The MCA (2005) requires the clinician in charge to make decisions based on what he or she feels is in the best interests of the patient. This is based not only on clinical factors but also on:

◆ the person's past and present wishes and feelings (and in particular, any relevant advance statement made by the person when they had capacity)

Box 4.5 Approaches to resolving disagreement between doctors and patients or those close to the them

- Discuss the issues with the patient or those close to them
- Explore the reasons for their views
- Re-assess benefits and harms
- Give due weight to patient's wishes and values
- If the decision is finely balanced the patient's wishes are usually determinative
- Having made the decision the reasons should be explained
- Consider a 2nd opinion or specialist advice, especially if:
  - You and the healthcare team have limited experience of a condition
  - You are uncertain about how to manage a patient's symptoms effectively
  - You are in doubt about the range of options, or the benefits, burdens, or risks of a particular option for the individual patient
  - There is a serious difference of opinion between you and the patient, within the healthcare team, or between the team and those close to a patient who lacks capacity to decide, about the preferred option for a patient's treatment and care.

- the beliefs and values likely to influence the person's decision if they had capacity
- other factors the person would be likely to consider if they were able to do so.

The Act requires discussion with those close to the patient when making the decision (24). However, those close to the patient are not the decision makers. In having this discussion there are relevant factors which the professional needs to consider:

- Relatives may not hold the same views as the patient, and if asked to make a decision the answer is likely to be what they would want for themselves
- They may not wish themselves to be seen as the person responsible for withdrawing treatments and so may be more proactive
- It is important to be aware of conflicts within families that might impair balanced decision making

The professional should make it clear that they are trying to find out what the patient would have wanted in these circumstances. If an understanding of the situation and a trusting relationship with the multidisciplinary team is established the family's emotional well being and the bereavement process that is to follow is likely to be less distressing.

Effective communication, providing regular updates on the situation and taking time to pass on decisions, may well prevent difficulties at a later stage. Blunt declarations to relatives that the decision is not theirs to make, or failure to discuss the relatives' suggestions, are unhelpful and potentially damaging. A careful exploration of their understanding of the situation, and of why they are requesting active treatment, usually helps to resolve most difficulties (Box 4.5).

How should an advance decision to refuse treatment or a legal proxy such as a lasting power of attorney affect the care of a patient on the LCP?

Advance decisions to refuse treatment (ADRT) or legal proxies such as lasting powers of attorney (LPA) should be recognized as a valid means by which patients can influence the treatments they receive when they are no longer competent to make decisions. They are legally binding in England and Wales (but note the further legal criteria that must be met for decisions that involve shortening life). Valid and applicable advance refusals are potentially binding in Scotland and Northern Ireland, although this has not yet been tested in the courts (4). Patients cannot use these tools to insist on additional treatments, although their views should always be considered. However, they can refuse interventions other than those relating to basic care.

The recognition in law given to these forms of advance care planning offer a number of benefits in resolving difficult end of life issues for the health care professional. They enable health care professionals to show respect for the patient's autonomy and to know what the patient would have perceived as being for their overall benefit—a decision which clinicians can sometimes find difficult. They can also help to relieve the family and carers from what they might perceive as an unwanted responsibility for advising over treatment decisions.

When presented with an ADRT health care professionals should clarify whether the patient was competent at the time of making the decision and whether they foresaw the situation they now find themselves in. The date of making the decision may also be relevant, as new developments may have occurred since that time which could alter the choices they would have made. A specific format is required and if the decision relates to a potentially life sustaining treatment then this needs specific mention (24,25).

A well prepared ADRT offers greater reassurance to the health care professional, especially if the contents go against medical advice. A number of organizations have prepared standard formats which may be useful (25). The
wording of the ADRT needs to strike a balance between being specific enough
to relate to the situation faced and yet broad enough to cover all scenarios that
may be encountered. They should be regularly reviewed and need to be readily
accessible. Relatives or carers need to know of their existence and ideally be
comfortable with their contents.

What is the role of an independent mental capacity advocate (IMCA) in decision making about the LCP?

When a patient is diagnosed as dying, the LCP process asks the professional to
consider the support of an IMCA as required.

NHS bodies must instruct and then take into account information from an
IMCA where finely balanced decisions are proposed about a 'serious medical
treatment,' where the person lacks capacity to make the decision and there are no
family or friends who are willing and able to support the person. Serious medical
treatment is that which involves giving new treatment, stopping treatment that
has already started or withholding treatment that could be offered (24).

Most patients do have people close to them who can act for them and in the
majority of cases the decision to commence the LCP is not finely balanced.
Therefore the need for an IMCA involvement is unusual in this decision making process. However, for patients who are unbefriended their role should be
considered.

Is it right that all patients should be offered a choice of dying in their preferred place?

To ask 'Would you like to die at home?' offers choice. This is not the same as
respecting the patient's autonomy. Explaining the key implications of such a
decision, establishing that the patient has capacity and has appreciated all the
important consequences, demonstrates respect for autonomy (26).

Health professionals have a responsibility to ensure decisions are based on
autonomous action by someone with capacity, who has full information and is
free from coercion, rather than being based merely on a simple choice. This
distinction is key in end of life decision-making.

If the patient makes an autonomous decision to die at home various considerations need to be balanced against each other:

+ The benefits to the patient of achieving their preferred place of death
+ The potential harms in terms of less specialist help or levels of care

- The need to use resources fairly
- The need to respect the autonomy of others, especially the main carers.

So, to answer the question, it is not necessarily right that patients should have a choice to die in their preferred place, but they should have their autonomous decision to die in their preferred place respected unless it is outweighed by considerations stemming from other moral principles.

Do patients have a right to die in their preferred place?

The answer to this question is similar to that of the previous one, in that the rights of one individual need to be balanced against the rights of any one else affected by this decision.

Is it justified to always discuss emotionally sensitive or distressing issues such as where people want to die?

The communication chapter will look at the skills required in these situations in more detail. Professionals should be able to assess the patient's information needs and preferences. By use of sensitive yet effective communication they should be able to establish the detail that patients are happy to discuss. Professionals should always attempt to raise important issues such as where a patient wants to die; omitting to do so fails to respect the autonomy of the patient.

If a patient is at home and refusing admission to hospital, yet the professional feels their care needs can be best met by admission; what is the right course of action?

We have considered how the four principles apply to the decision making process in choosing the place of care. In this situation assessment is required to ensure the patient is making an autonomous decision. If so, then this needs to be weighed up against the benefits and harms to them and a consideration made of the resources required. Consideration should also be given to the views of those close to the patient, on whom the burden of care falls. If all necessary steps have been taken to provide support, then should this burden still be too great there would be a reason to deny the patient the wish to die at home. Respect for the patient's autonomous decision is dependent on their also respecting the autonomy of others.

Finally, consideration is required as to whether the professional is basing their assessment on their own perspective rather than being sufficiently empathic to enable them to see the patient's perspective. In assessing the right action it is the patient's interpretation that ultimately counts, however far this may be from our own as professionals.

Further resources

E learning in end of life care: http://www.e-lfh.org.uk/projects/e-elca/index.html

General Medical Council: http://www.gmc-uk.org/

Association for Palliative Medicine: http://www.palliative-medicine.org/

The gold standards framework: http://www.goldstandardsframework.nhs.uk/

The Marie Curie Palliative Care Institute: www.mcpcil.org.uk

National Council for Palliative Care: http://www.ncpc.org.uk/

British Heart Foundation: http://www.bhf.org.uk

National End of Life Care Programme: http://www.endoflifecare.nhs.uk/eolc/

Resuscitation Council: www.resus.org.uk

Mental Capacity Act: www.publicguardian.gov.uk/mca/mca.htm

Independent Mental Capacity Advocate Service: www.dh.gov.uk/imca

Adults with incapacity act (Scotland): http://www.scotland.gov.uk/Topics/Justice/law/awi

Mental Welfare Commission for Scotland: www.mwcscot.org.uk/newpublications/good_
practice_guidance.asp

References

1 Beauchamp TL, and Childress JF. (2008). *Principles of biomedical ethics.* Oxford University Press, New York.

2 Seale C. End-of-life decisions in the UK involving medical practitioners. *Palliat Med* 2009;**23**:198–204.

3 General medical council. *End of life care: Flow chart for decision making when patients may lack capacity* http://www.gmc-uk.org/guidance/ethical_guidance/6997.asp (accessed 28 June 2010)

4 General Medical Council. *Treatment and Care Towards the End of Life: Good Practice in Decision Making.* GMC, London 2010.

5 Re B Adult: refusal of medical treatment (2002) High court ruling, 2 All ER 449.

6 British Medical Association. *Withholding and withdrawing life prolonging treatment.* 3rd Ed. BMA, London 2007.

7 Sandroni C, Nolan J, Cavallaro F, Antonelli M. In-hospital cardiac arrest: incidence, prognosis and possible measures to improve survival. *Intensive Care Med* 2007;**33**(2):237–45.

8 Nolan JP, Laver SR, Welch CA et al. Outcome following admission to UK intensive care units after cardiac arrest: a secondary analysis of the ICNARC Case Mix Programme Database. *Anaesthesia.* 2007;**62**(12):1207–16.

9 Diem SJ, Lantos JD, Tulsky JA. Cardiopulmonary Resuscitation on Television— Miracles and Misinformation *N Engl J Med* 1996; **334**(24):1578–82.

10 Gordon PN, Williamson S, Lawler PG. As seen on TV: observational study of cardiopulmonary resuscitation in British television medical dramas. *BMJ* 1998;**317**(7161):780–3.

11 Joint Working Party between the National Council for Hospice and Specialist Palliative Care Services and the Ethics Committee of the Association for Palliative Medicine of

Great Britain and Ireland. *Ethical decision making: Cardiopulmonary resuscitation (CPR) for people who are terminally ill.* National Council for Hospital and Specialist Palliative Care Services, London, 2002.

12 British Medical Association, Resuscitation Council (UK), Royal College of Nursing. *Decisions relating to cardiopulmonary resuscitation: a joint statement from the British Medical Association, the Resuscitation Council (UK) and the Royal College of Nursing.* London: BMA, 2007.

13 British Heart Foundation. *Implantable cardioverter defibrillators in patients who are reaching the end of life.* London BHF 2007.

14 Good P, Cavenagh J, Mather M, Ravenscroft P. *Medically assisted hydration for adult palliative care patients.* Cochrane Database of Systematic Reviews 2008, Issue **2**. Art. No.: CD006273. DOI: 10.1002/14651858.CD006273.pub2.

15 Campbell C, Partridge R. *Artificial Nutrition and Hydration–Guidance in end of life care for adults.* National Council for Palliative Care and Association for Palliative Medicine, London. May 2007.

16 Lennard-Jones JE. Giving or withholding fluid and nutrients: ethical and legal aspects. *J R Coll Physicians* 1999;**33**:39–45.

17 Good P, Cavenagh J, Mather M, Ravenscroft P. *Medically assisted nutrition for palliative care in adult patients.* Cochrane Database of Systematic Reviews 2008, Issue 4. Art. No.: CD006274. DOI: 10.1002/14651858.CD006274.pub2.

18 Estfan B, Mahmoud F, Shaheen P et al. Respiratory function during parenteral opioid titration for cancer pain. *Palliat Med* 2007;**21**:81–86.

19 George R, Regnard C. Lethal opioids or dangerous prescribers. *Palliat Med* 2007;**21**(2):77–80.

20 Sykes NP, Thorns A. The use of opioids and sedatives at the end of life in palliative care. *Lancet Oncol* 2003;**4**:312–8.

21 Fainsinger RL, Waller A, Bercovici M, Bengston K, Landman W, Hosking M, et al. A multicentre international study of sedation for uncontrolled symptoms in terminally ill patients. *Palliat. Med* 2000;**14**(4), 257–65.

22 The Director of Public Prosecutions. *Policy for Prosecutors in respect of Cases of Encouraging or Assisting Suicide.* Crown Prosecution Service. London. February 2010.

23 Barker I. Prosecuting cases of assisted suicide. *MDU Journal* 2009;**25**(2):8.

24 Department for Constitutional Affairs. *Code of Practice Mental Capacity Act.* 2005, DCA, London.

25 *Advance decisions to refuse treatment* available from www.adrtnhs.co.uk (accessed on 16 December 2009).

26 Downie R, Randall F. Choice and responsibility in the NHS. *Clin Med* 2008;**8**:182–5.

Chapter 5

Communication in care of the dying

Susie Wilkinson

A major component of the successful delivery of the Liverpool Care Pathway for the Dying Patient (LCP) is communication; communication with patients and their carers. Communication has been defined in a variety of ways. For the purpose of this chapter communication is defined as 'an interchange of thoughts, feelings, and opinions among individuals. Verbal communication is effective when it satisfies basic desires for recognition, participation, and self-realization by direct personal contact between persons' (1).

The importance of effective communication skills within healthcare is well documented (2–4). Patients and their relatives regard good communication with health professionals as a high priority. Ineffective communication leaves people feeling anxious, frustrated, and dissatisfied (5,6). In the interests of patients' safety it is also essential that healthcare professionals can communicate with patients (7). Whether communication is verbal or non-verbal it occurs during every encounter between individuals. When communicating distressing and complex information, as is often required when implementing the LCP, healthcare professionals should have enhanced skills, or be supported by someone who has those skills, as the use of any tool such as the LCP is only as effective as the professionals using it. Health professionals may in the future also have to demonstrate competence in communicating with patients (5).

There is a general assumption that effective communication is achieved when open two-way communication takes place, and patients are informed about the nature of their illness and treatment and are encouraged to express their anxieties and emotions. This view assumes that open communication, full information about a disease and its prognosis, has benefits for all patients. Many health professionals and relatives fear that being open and honest with patients will result in psychological distress. There is little evidence to substantiate this view and what is evident is that if patients receive ambiguous or conflicting information this is likely to increase their psychological distress (6,8). However, people need to be given the opportunity to consider what care they wish to receive at the end of their lives based on the best available information about what may lie ahead of them and what services are available. It also needs to be recognized that some people will not wish to confront their own mortality and will not wish to enter into conversations either with their families or with health and social care staff. If this is their choice, it should be respected (9).

The importance of supportive communication was poignantly highlighted by an American oncology nurse dying of breast cancer. Days before her death she completed a paper, which was delivered posthumously by her husband. Bushkin wrote:

> There are so many questions, concerns, and problems to face in the lightening ball mirror. To overcome the sense of powerlessness the traveller (ie patient) runs through a maze seeking someone who might actually listen to their pleas for help, someone who actually knows that the traveller is there. The question of being heard and having one's questions answered is a perpetual source of frustration. In the absence of recognition the traveller feels alone and at the mercy of those who do not hear (10).

To avoid the difficulties Buskin described the key for all health professionals is to be able to asses the patient's communication and information needs and tailor their communication to meet those needs. All relevant staff involved with end of life care need to be able to undertake a comprehensive assessment of the needs and preferences of a person relating to their physical, social and occupational, psychological, and spiritual wellbeing. Also the assessment needs to be interactive, non-mechanistic and over a period of time (9).

In end of life care the challenges are even greater than usual because of the expectation that health professionals will be able to discuss, support and cope with patients facing death.

Healthcare professionals are generally trained to be clinical and practical and their communication skills instinctively follow that route and deal with patients' difficulties at that practical level. What patients and relatives also need at the end of life is communication at a more emotional level which acknowledges their difficult and stressful situation. Health professionals' psychosocial skills have been shown to determine patients' satisfaction, compliance, and health outcomes, even to the extent that if health professionals explore patients' concerns and feelings even when their concerns cannot be resolved a significant fall in patient anxiety levels is noted (11).

Health professionals' communication skills do not reliably improve with experience. It is also necessary to learn and understand certain skills and knowledge, and be able to explore attitudes (12). Furthermore, insufficient training in communication skills can contribute to stress and burnout in healthcare professionals (13).

There is good evidence that communication skills in cancer care and heart disease can be taught and sustained over a period of time. (14–19). Importantly it is now recognized that all health and social care workers need some training to ensure that they are able to communicate effectively with people who are dying and their carers about issues surrounding end of life care (9).

The chapter therefore proposes to raise awareness of the communication skills, assessment skills, and strategies to handle the many difficult situations that frequently arise when caring for patients and their relatives at the end of a patient's life. The strategies described are not exclusive but are the most frequent difficulties encountered by participants undertaking an advanced communication skills training course for senior healthcare professionals in cancer and palliative care (8).

What are the skills that facilitate communication?

Patients are more likely to disclose their concerns to those professionals who demonstrate that they are prepared to listen and are open to discussion (20). This involves the use of verbal and non-verbal communication skills which facilitate the patient and their relatives to discuss their worries or concerns.

Non-verbal communication plays a large part in portraying how patients feel. Health professionals' non-verbal behaviours often demonstrate to patients a commitment to listening to their concerns. The importance of adopting good non-verbal behaviours cannot be over-emphasized and are briefly described in Table 5.1.

In caring for dying patients, there are vital verbal skills to be adopted. Verbal communication can be divided into two parts; the language, ie the actual words used and paralanguage, ie how it is said, for example, the tone of voice, volume, pitch, clarity, and rate.

Table 5.2 describes the main verbal skills with examples that facilitate good communication. However some behaviours that often are thought by health professionals to be facilitating for patients, in fact hinder communication and can prevent patients and relatives disclosing their concerns.

Blocking tactics that can hinder communication

Blocking tactics were first noted by Quint (21) who observed health professionals interacting with patients with breast cancer. Over twenty years later Wilkinson (2) described a more comprehensive account of the behaviours that were still being used to block communication. Most of the participants involved in the study were unaware that the behaviours they were using hindered communication. These behaviours are described in Table 5.3.

Table 5.1 Adoptive behaviours of professionals, patients, and relatives

Personal space	Area around the body, which, if intruded by some people and cultures, leaves one feeling uncomfortable. It is important to sit down squarely in relation to the patient to allow all aspects of communication to be seen; paralinguistic, such as sighs, grunts, and non-verbal bodily communication. It is also necessary to lean towards the patient to encourage them and make them feel more understood
Facial expressions	Display emotions, which may conflict or support the spoken word, ie nodding, agreeing or disagreeing, frown lines, position of the eye brows and eye lids, size of pupils
Eye contact	Important in building satisfying relationships; should be reasonably sustained. Ratio of contact professional : patient = 1: 1. Avoidance can signal discomfort or disinterest
Posture	Demonstrates attitudes, emotions, and mood; supports or conflicts the spoken word. Open position to be adopted in relation to the patient. A 'closed' position, such as crossing both arms and legs, can convey a defensive feeling
Gestures	Illustrates speech, expresses emotions, ie raising a finger, increased hand movements indicating anxiety, minimal hand movements indicating depression
Touching	Helps develop a caring relationship; expresses emotion. Dying patients often feel the need for physical contact with carers; holding hands provides physical expression to the personal relationship

Table 5.2 Verbal skills

Listening	An active skill that requires great concentration if the patient's cues are to be addressed	
Silences	Allows both parties to think and assimilate what has been said	
Acknowledgement	Utterances that indicate the patient is being heard and taken note of	*Mmmh, uuh, yes.*
Encouragement	More active than acknowledgement. Important in the maintenance of interaction. Actively shows interest and understanding, encourages the patient to continue	*Really, that is important, please do go on.*
Picking up cues	Patients drop subtle hints or verbal or non-verbal cues of concerns. The skill lies in being able to pick up on these	Q: *How are you today?* A: *I'm fine really, **it's the family that have been upsetting me.*** The cue is highlighted.

Table 5.2 *(Cont'd)* Verbal skills

Reflection	Encourages discussion around a problem raised and in depth/further analysis.	Q: *The family have been upsetting you, in what way have they been upsetting you?*
Open questioning	Provide room for patients to express themselves. Elicit feelings	*How do you feel today? How have you been sleeping?*
Clarification	Questions that ensure the patient's meaning is understood. Enables more detailed information on problems or concerns to emerge	A: *I'm feeling non-plussed* Q: *What do you mean by that?* Or A: *That will be it.* Q: *What exactly do you mean by that will be it?*
Empathy	Statements which demonstrate understanding from the patients' point of view. Encourages the patient to go into more depth	*It sounds as if things have been very hard for you lately.* Or *From what you have said, I get the feeling that you have been feeling very low.*
Confrontation/ challenge	Questions or statements that challenge discrepancies in what patients say	*You've said you are feeling fine and have no worries, but you have just said that you are feeling anxious. Can you tell me a bit more about this?*
Information giving	Patients should only be given required information. Assessment of their informational needs should be done prior to release of information. Patients are only able to retain small amounts of information at a time; this needs to be given slowly, without jargon or technical terms in small chunks, and then their understanding of the information need to be checked.	*I have given you a great deal of information. Can you tell me exactly what you have understood?*

The reason for describing these behaviours is because many health professionals have adopted them by habit without realizing the effects. This is not to say they should never be used. There are situations when they are used as protection for our own emotional stability in an often very stressful area of care. However, in order to help patients, their use should be minimized.

Once the basic communication skills have been mastered they need to be put into action to address the situations that arise when patients are supported by the LCP.

Table 5.3 Blocking behaviours

Normalizing	Automatic placatory comments that convey either a lack of understanding from the patient's point of view, or that the patient's experiences are not unique or important. These comments simply shift the focus away from the patient. Comments such as this make it very difficult for patients to voice their fears or worries further.	*Everyone feels frightened of dying it is normal*
False or premature reassurance	Remarks and comments made to the patient which provide a false or premature sense of reassurance and are more positive than the situation warrants	*You won't have any pain because we will give you pain killers*
Inappropriate advice	Advice which encourages a decision to be made by the patient by imposing one's own opinions and solutions, as opposed to assisting the patient with exploration of ways of arriving at a conclusion	patient: *I don't know whether to take this sedative* professional: *Well I would if it was me*
Leading questions	A question is asked in such a way as to predetermine a particular response from a patient	*You are looking fine, you must be feeling fine?*
Closed questions	Type of question that can restrict the range of possible responses from a patient, encouraging a monosyllabic 'yes' or 'no' as opposed to inviting discussion or expression of feeling	*Any problems with your sleep?* as opposed to *How are you sleeping?*
Multiple questioning	Questions can be asked in a confusing torrent without pausing for a reply to each	*How do you feel? Have you any pain? Did you sleep well?'*
Passing the buck	Deflecting the patient to another colleague when asked a specific and uncomfortable question instead of exploring the concerns behind the question first	patient: *I don't feel as if I am getting any better.* professional: *Ask the doctor about this when you next see him.*
Requesting an explanation	The analysis is passed back to the patient by asking for an explanation of feelings or actions, sometimes with an intimidating and stark 'why'?	patient: *I didn't sleep last night.* professional: *Why didn't you sleep?*
Approving/ agreeing	Remarks and opinions can shift the focus to the professionals' own feelings and values. This imposes upon and restricts the patients' own free expression	patient: *My family have been worrying me.* professional: *I think you need to stop worrying about your family and concentrate on yourself.*
Defensive behaviours	When a patient becomes angry or worried, excuses are made rather than allowing the patient to explore and express his feelings and opinions	patient: *I'm really worried about dying.* professional: *Oh the chaplain is really good, he is the expert in this area.*

Table 5.3 *(Cont'd)* Blocking behaviours

Shifting the focus to relatives	In discussions with the patient, focus can be shifted from their problems to the relative and thus emphasis is removed from how the patient feels, to how his relatives feel or think	patient: *I think I'm going to find it hard going into the hospice.* professional: *What does your wife think about it?*
Selective attention to cue	When cues or questions are raised, a response is selected to address the physical rather than the emotional aspects	patient: *My pain has gone, but I'm feeling very low.* professional: *I'm pleased your pain has gone.*
Jollying along	Some bright and cheerful placatory remarks or comments are merely glossing over real issues in the hope that the patient will feel better. These in fact make the patient feel uneasy in stating their true feelings	*Don't look so glum! It's a gorgeous day outside. Give me a smile.*
Irrelevant chit chat:	Personal irrelevant chit chat removes the focus of the interaction from the patient and their concerns, back to the professional.	

Are the patient and their family aware of the patient's deteriorating condition?

Interviewing and assessment skills form the basis of all communication interaction (19). The uniqueness of each patient can only be recognized by carrying out a comprehensive assessment which addresses the patient's agenda (19). Assessment is gathering information about the patient from the patient's perspective. It is not, as some health professionals believe, just giving information. The time and place for giving information is after an assessment when all the patient's concerns and informational needs have been established. Some health professionals undervalue the role of an assessment and see it merely as a form filling exercise (20). Assessment however is possibly the most vital part of care as without an accurate assessment it is not possible to plan good quality individualized care. There are nine key areas for a comprehensive patient assessment (Table 5.4) however, when implementing the LCP it may not be appropriate to assess all areas comprehensively. According to the National Hospital audit report, the patients' insight into their diagnosis was only achieved for 50 per cent of patients, and recognition of dying in 40 per cent of patients, indicating that staff still find this area of assessment very challenging (22).

The patient assessment

To assess the patient's insight of their diagnosis or prognosis, the discussion needs to be carefully organized in terms of setting adequate time aside;

Table 5.4 Key areas for a comprehensive patient assessment

---

1. Introduction
   - Establish initial rapport by introducing self, state name and role, and ask for patient's preferred form of address
   - Negotiate length of time required for assessment. Briefly outline of the purpose of this task
   - Attend to 'patient's agenda' and ascertain if they have anything in particular that they wish to discuss

2. Patient's understanding of their admission/visit

3. Patient's understanding and history of their present illness

4. Patient's awareness of their diagnosis/prognosis

5. Patient's history of previous illness if appropriate

6. Physical assessment

7. Social/occupational assessment

8. Psychological/spiritual assessment

9. Closure of assessment
   Summarize patient's main concerns or worries
   - Check if anything has been missed by asking a screening question such as; 'is there anything else that you want to tell me about before we move on to looking at how we might help?'
   - Ask the patient to prioritize their concerns or worries, so that the most important ones are addressed first
   - Thank the patient for sharing their concerns
   - Inform patient of how and who to contact for help if it is required.

---

agreeing the venue; and giving the patient the option to have a relative(s) present, if they wish, who may provide valuable support.

The venue should be a quiet and private setting away from interruptions and distractions such as telephone calls, bleeps, and uninvited visitors. This is to ensure privacy for the patient and relatives to encourage an open dialogue. However, it is recognized that in some care settings (such as a main ward within a hospital) it is sometimes difficult to provide privacy. In such cases, make the situation as private as possible by screening an area off and informing staff of the intended discussions. The amount and level of information regarding the patient's diagnosis and prognosis, needs to be guided by both verbal and non-verbal cues from the patient.

To gain the patient's confidence and trust, initially it is important to gather information from the patient themselves. Let the patient if possible tell their story and establish what their understanding is; not just what the doctor has said. A useful framework that can be helpful for this assessment is the ICE framework (23) which ascertains the patient's:

- **Ideas** What the patient believes, their thoughts and feelings about their condition .
- **Concerns** What are the patient's particular concerns or worries at this time
- **Expectations** What are the patient's thoughts for the future? What are they hoping for, expecting, and what would they like to happen?

Examples of the kind of open questions that could be used to implement this framework are:

- Can you tell me in your own words what you understand about your illness?
- How did you feel when the doctor told you about your illness?
- How do you feel things are going for you at the moment/just now?
- What thoughts have you been having/had about your illness?
- What are your particular concerns or worries at the moment?
- How have you been physically?
- What would you like to know about your illness that might help you understand your present situation?
- What has been going through your mind about the future?

Establish with whom the patient has a meaningful relationship and the extent of support from the relationship:

- How is your family coping with your illness?
- Which family member would you like me to talk with?
- What concerns do you have regarding your family at this time?

Establish the patient's present mood, in terms of how the illness is affecting them. Pick up on any cues as to how the patient has been feeling in terms of anxiety and depression:

- How have you been feeling in your spirits?
- What has been the most difficult part of this illness?
- What is the worst thing that could happen?
- Is there anything in particular that makes you feel anxious or worried?

Establish whether the patient has any faith adherence, or wishes to be referred to a health care chaplain or faith leader. Further details and suggested questions for a spiritual/religious assessment are addressed in Chapter 6.

Once an assessment of the patient has been made it is vital that details of the assessment are fully documented. Thirty one per cent of the patients' insights of their condition awareness were not documented on the recent LCP audit (22). Documentation is vital in order that all the multidisciplinary team are aware of the patient's condition, thoughts, and beliefs.

Handling difficult questions

Some patients in the final stages of their life are aware of the significance of certain symptoms, such as increasing weakness and weight loss that confirms the fact that death is approaching and that they are dying, and often pose questions like, 'Am I dying?' or 'I'm not going to get better, am I?' or 'I am not going to make it, am I?' Healthcare professionals often find such questions very difficult to handle for fear of upsetting the patients. Figure 5.1 outlines a structure of a possible way to handle such difficult questions.

What has happened for the patient to ask the question?

The patient obviously has been thinking about the issue, otherwise they would not have asked the question. It is therefore necessary to explore the patient's thought processes, guiding them with a question such as, 'I'm happy to talk to you about the question you have asked but it would just help me if you could tell me what, if anything, has prompted you to ask me this question today?' This is particularly important if the question is posed in an obscure way such as 'I am not going to make it, am I?' In this situation it is important not to assume that you know the meaning of the question. Check with the patient by reflection and clarification, for example 'When you say you are not going to

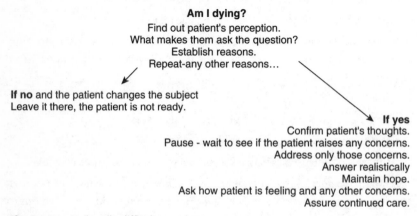

Fig. 5.1 How to handle difficult questions.

make it, what exactly do you mean by that?' The patient may respond that for one or two reasons they feel that they are not getting better.

Checking readiness for receiving bad news

How the patient is likely to cope psychologically with bad news can sometimes be judged by first establishing whether the patient is ready to receive confirmation of their own thoughts. Some patients ask a question and then wish that they had not, particularly if they perceive the news will be bad. To guard against this in some situations, particularly if you are a member of the multidisciplinary team and not the doctor, it is sometimes a good idea to give the patient a second chance by asking them, 'You've told me one or two reasons why you feel that you are not getting any better, or you feel that you are dying, are there any other reasons?' The patient now has two options. They can either say that there are some additional reasons for feeling they are deteriorating or dying, or they can simply change the subject, thus demonstrating that they are not actually ready to receive bad news at that point in time.

Confirming bad news

When the patient gives other reasons as to why they feel they are dying, this is a good indication that they are aware of their situation. In this instance there is only one path open; to confirm to the patient that their thoughts are correct. For example, 'It appears from what you've said that you feel that you are dying and yes, I'm afraid I think your thoughts are correct, and I think you are dying.'

A typical reaction from health professionals on having broken bad news is a desire to make the situation 'better' for the patient by giving information on how symptoms for example can be controlled. This can result in actually giving reassurance for symptoms that the patient may not have thought about giving them more worries. It is therefore necessary to wait until the patient raises their concerns or worries, and then address those concerns alone. Common fears and concerns are listed in Box 5.1.

Dealing with patients' questions realistically

If a patient asks 'How long have I got' establish in the first instance if there is a reason for asking that question. It could be because they have not made a will or they are trying to establish if they will live long enough to enjoy a particular birthday or other celebration.

Try whenever possible to answer patients' questions realistically. If the patient asks if they will experience any pain, rather than saying, 'Oh, no, you won't have any pain, we will look after that'; it is preferable to highlight to the

Box 5.1 Common fears and concerns for some dying patients

How long have I got?

How will I die, what will happen?

Where will I die?

Will I be in pain?

Will I choke?

Will I be alone?

Will I be unable to breathe?

What happens after I die?

Unfinished business; things to do, e.g. making a will.

patient that they must tell the staff if they ever have any pain; let the patient know that there are many different methods of controlling pain; and reassure the patient that you will do your best and hopefully they will not be in pain. This kind of response is the one that helps to maintain patients' hope. By indicating that while it may not be possible to effect the outcome of their situation, there is still a great deal of care that can be given to alleviate distressing symptoms. At this point if the use of the LCP to support the care being given is to be implemented it would be appropriate to discuss this with the patient.

Dealing with uncertainty

Difficult questions such as 'How long have I got before I die' often leads to uncertainty for patients which can be very challenging for them or their family. The use of empathy is of great value in these situations. Firstly acknowledge the difficulty of the predicament for example 'I appreciate how difficult this situation is for you when we cannot give you a definitive answer. It must be very hard for you.' Then invite the patient to talk about how they feel about the uncertainty and what you have discussed and any other concerns they have that they would like addressed. If there are no other concerns at that present moment in time, convey to the patient that any future concerns can be discussed at a later date and you and the team will be there for ongoing support. Documentation that these important discussions have taken place is vital.

Breaking bad news of a deteriorating condition

In certain situations patients never ask difficult questions such as 'Am I dying' and it becomes necessary for health professionals to break the news of a deteriorating condition, particularly if after discussions with the multidisciplinary team treatments have to be withheld or withdrawn, and the focus of care is to change, and/or the LCP is to be implemented to support care. Bad news is bad news. It is not possible to soften the impact, but the way in which bad news is given can help the patient's adjustment to a deteriorating condition. The Healthcare Commission report identified that most complaints around communication were related to how news was broken to patients and relatives when the patient was dying (6). For many patients it is not what is said but how it is said, including the manner in which it is said. The key is to slow down the speed of transition from a perception of being ill to the realization that death could be close. Preparation in these situations is vital. The place and sufficient time needs to be planned as well as making sure all relevant details are to hand and if appropriate involve a relative or friend. Box 5.2 could be a useful framework for breaking bad news of a deteriorating condition.

Begin by sign posting to the patient that there is something important you would like to discuss with them. This is often interpreted by patients as a warning shot.

The task of breaking bad news is often made less difficult if the patient's perceptions of how they feel they are doing is established, e.g. 'It would be helpful if you could tell me how you feel things are going at the moment', or 'What has been going through your mind about how you have been recently?' If the patient indicates they are aware of their deteriorating condition, the strategy for confirming their thoughts as used above for handling a difficult question can be used. If however the patient seems unaware of their deterioration find out how much the patient would like to know about their condition.

Box 5.2 Breaking bad news of a deteriorating condition

- Establish what the patient already knows
- Establish how much the patient wants to know
- Give a warning shot
- Break the bad news using simple and clear language
- Pause and wait for a response
- Assess and focus on the patient's feelings
- Encourage the patient to express their concerns
- Check patient's understanding and invite questions
- Develop a plan of care and discuss future care with the patient
- Assure follow-up

'How much information about your condition would be helpful for you to have?' Once this is ascertained give the patient a warning shot, e.g. 'I am afraid things are not going too well.' Wait for a response as the patient may confirm that they are aware things are not going well. If not, break the bad news using simple and clear language, e.g. 'I am afraid to say that your condition has been getting worse and causing us concern (give examples of worsening symptoms or results of tests if appropriate) and we think you are dying'. Pause and wait for a response and focus initially only on the patient's responses or questions. Assess and focus on how the patient is feeling about what they have been told. Encourage the patient to express their concerns. If the patient is happy to continue it may be an appropriate time to discuss sensitively ongoing care which may involve where a patient would like to die, and or, withdrawing or withholding treatments (see Chapter 4) emphasizing that with the implementation of the LCP (if being used) ongoing care will focus more on comfort and maintaining dignity.

Communicating with relatives

As patients deteriorate, relatives too need the opportunity to ask questions about the significance of the patient's deterioration and be given appropriate explanations. If the patient's deterioration has been discussed with the patient on their own with the patient's permission the situation should then be discussed with the relatives. If the patient is unconscious or unable to communicate, the relatives' awareness of the patient's diagnosis and recognition of dying will need to be established and, if necessary, the relatives will need to be informed of the patient's deteriorating condition. The framework in Box 5.2 'Breaking bad news of a deteriorating condition' can be very usefully adapted for discussions with relatives. It may also be a pertinent time to discuss (if appropriate) the implementation of the LCP with relatives and give them the information sheet which asks them to document any questions that they think of. Such a conversation reinforces that the patient is reaching the end of their life. At this time it is also important to identify how the family wish to be informed about the patient's death, for example who should be contacted should a further deterioration occur. For many relatives, being present at the time of death is very important. It is therefore necessary to establish at what stage the family would like to be called in should the patient's condition deteriorate and where and when they wish to be contacted, ie night or day or at work.

Some relatives may wish to stay overnight with the patient and, depending on the conditions within the organization, this will determine whether it is possible or not. It is common for relatives who stay overnight with the patient to feel a compulsion to stay by the patient's bedside constantly. Thus, they become anxious about leaving and often need encouragement from staff to take some time out.

Many dying patients, increasingly dependent upon professionals and relatives, convey feelings of extreme fatigue, and although they may wish for relatives to be present, they feel a dilemma of being over-visited but yet are unable to express their feelings without being insensitive to the needs of their family.

Thus, sensitive communications, often on behalf of the patient, should take place and agreements reached to set limits on the number and frequency of agreed visitors. One way forward may be the suggestion of a visiting rota to enable both patient and visitors to get some rest.

If the relatives are with the patient when they die, many are often not aware death has actually occurred. Therefore they need to be taken aside and informed sensitively and with empathy that the patient has died. The words death and died should always be used as this is highlighted as one of the goals of the LCP. Euphemisms such as passed away and passed on should not be used as these just reinforce the taboo of talking about death and dying that exists in modern society. An anecdotal example illustrates how if the word death or dying is not used relatives can be confused. A patient following a road traffic accident was admitted to A and E. Resuscitation was taking place when the relatives arrived and this was explained to the relatives. When resuscitation failed the doctor informed the relatives who were in a state of shock that they were sorry they had 'lost him'. The relatives, not realizing the patient had died went for a cup of tea and returned an hour later to ask if the patient had been found. This very unfortunate incident clearly reinforces how important it is to use the correct words when communicating with relatives.

Handling feelings and emotions

Often when patients or relatives have been told bad news they experience emotions such as distress or anger. A strategy for handling distress is shown in Box 5.3.

If people become very distressed and cry, acknowledge that they are upset by saying, for example, 'I can see that you are really upset by what I have just said and I would like you to tell me if there are any specific issues or feelings that you would like to share with me.' This kind of approach usually facilitates the patient to actually talk about their upset.

It is then important to accept what the patient says empathically. Summarize how they feel, for example, 'You sound as if you are upset because . . . and I appreciate how upsetting this must be for you.' Empathy facilitates the patient to discuss their distress. Empathy is a skill that is not widely used but it offers patients very gently an opportunity to talk (3). Sometimes patients prefer not to

Box 5.3 Handling distress

Recognition	Evidence verbally/non-verbally of distress. *I can see how upset you are*
Acknowledgement	*I appreciate just how upsetting this must be for you*
Permission and Understanding	*If it is alright with you it would be very helpful if you could share with me if there is something in particular that is upsetting you as I appreciate this is a very difficult situation*
Acceptance using empathy	*It sounds as if you are upset because . . .*
Alteration (if appropriate)	Removal of upset

discuss their distress and they will say so and their decision must be respected. Empathy is the ability to perceive the meaning and feelings of another person and communicate that feeling to the other person (24). There are many situations in end of life care when patients and relatives realize that health professionals cannot solve their problems, but having the opportunity to voice their concerns maintains hope, and to do this sensitively with empathy is necessary.

Hope is a coping strategy used by those confronted with a serious illness. As Bushkin (10) highlighted, hope is extremely important. Hope is a difficult concept to measure, and to date a qualitative rather than quantitative research approach has been used in the majority of studies. Communication behaviours clearly influence patients' hope and Koopmeiners et al. (25) identified that taking time to talk, giving information when requested, being friendly, polite, helpful, and honest as well as just being there, demonstrating caring behaviours were the most important influences on patients' maintenance of hope in a palliative care setting.

In many end of life situations patients or their relatives become very frustrated or angry that things are not going as they had hoped. Sometimes the expression of anger can signify that the person is finding their situation very difficult to cope with. Other times their anger may be justifiable. The main aim in attempting to handle anger is to allow the person to communicate what is making them so angry to diffuse the situation. Box 5.4 describes steps that can be tried in these highly emotive situations.

Communicating with families who want to protect patients from the truth

Many relatives wish to protect their loved ones from receiving bad news, and ask health professionals not to disclose bad news. To overcome this situation it

Box 5.4 Handling anger

- Do not say 'calm down'
- Ignore sarcasms and put downs that would lead to more anger and argument
- Try not to take anger personally
- Acknowledge and recognize the anger by saying 'I can see you are very angry'
- Try to move the person from an emotional state to a more rational state
- Give permission to be angry by saying 'I really want to hear what you are angry about and what you have to say'
- If appropriate sensitively ask 'but can you please speak more quietly so that I can hear what you have to say'
- Establish facts, listen to the story, get as much information as possible
- Concentrate on the person and their stress/feelings
- Maintain eye contact
- Recap and summarize to be clear of facts
- Try to negotiate a solution
- 'What can I do to help' or 'Lets work on this together'
- Take action if appropriate.

is necessary to gain the relatives' confidence so that they do not think the patient would be unilaterally approached and told that they are dying. One way of coping with this situation is shown in Box 5.5. It is vital initially to accept what the relative has requested by saying 'I can entirely agree with what you are saying, but can I ask you though how you are?' and find out how the relative feels they are coping and communicating with their loved one. This often highlights that relatives are under considerable strain. Keeping the truth from the patient is stressful. It is sometimes appropriate to actually highlight that collusion can strain a relationship.

Once the relatives' feelings have been explored, the reasons for them not wanting to be truthful with the patient need to be discussed. Whatever the reason it is important that these reasons are supported. The next step is to ask the relative whether the patient has in fact asked any questions about their illness. In most cases the patient will have asked some questions. It is therefore vital to suggest that because the patient has asked some questions it indicates that they may have some idea of their true condition.

Box 5.5 Collusion

- Focus on how the relatives are feeling
- Their reasons for not wanting to be truthful
- The strain on their relationship
- Support their reasons
- Assess any patient questions to the relatives
- Suggest a window on knowledge
- Ask for permission to assess the patient
- Reassure no telling
- But confirmation will be given to the patient if necessary.

The relative still needs reassurance that the patient's condition will not just be divulged to them, but it needs to be pointed out that, as a member of the multidisciplinary team looking after them, you will need to find out how the patient is feeling and whether they have any concerns or worries to discuss. It is also important to 'flag up' to the relative that, should in the course of discussions the patient disclose that they know that they are dying and are able to substantiate their reasons as to why they think they are dying, it would only be fair and ethical to confirm the patient's own assessment of the situation. If the patient does disclose that they are aware of their true condition, it is then necessary to make contact with the family and inform them that whilst talking to the patient they raised concerns about their for example weight loss and increased breathlessness and whether that meant they were dying, and that you responded to this question by confirming to the patient that they were correct in their belief. Frequently relatives are concerned that the patient will 'fall apart' or be very distressed. It is therefore important to stress to the relatives (if appropriate) that the patient was naturally upset but was relieved that they now know. In some cases this serves to enable the patient and their family to share feelings at a very difficult time.

Cultural issues in communication

In a multi-cultural society communication difficulties may arise with patients when they and their families are from ethnic groups where English is not their first language. These communication difficulties are difficult for staff, as they are unable to accurately assess the patient's understanding of what is being said. The patient may appear to confirm his understanding of what is being discussed with an affirmative gesture, such as a nod. However, this may not be a response to the discussions taking place but may be an instinctive reaction to the patient's embarrassment in failing to comprehend the details of the conversation.

It is therefore desirable that every health care organization has easy access to a panel of competent interpreters from whom support is readily available. They often can with close guidance and support, enter into a dialogue with the patient, assess the patient's level of understanding of the present situation, and address his concerns and anxieties.

Observation of the body language and extent of dialogue between the interpreter and the patient is crucial as this can be a reasonable indicator that the interpretations given are those from the patient and not merely perceptions of the interpreter.

An effective interpretation of the situation is fundamental in enabling the patient and family to become fully cognizant of the patient's deterioration and treatment management. This also provides an opportunity for them to ask questions and express their anxieties, concerns, and fears.

In the case where an uncommon language is encountered, and ready access to an interpreter is not available, contact can be made with the appropriate Embassy or High Commission who may be able to advise on appropriate action or supply a suitable contact. This may be time-consuming and the patient may have to wait for some time before a suitable interpreter is located. Therefore other means of communication, such as basic sign language may be adopted to help elicit crucial information to alleviate the patient's and family's anxieties and reassure them that their situation is being addressed and managed. Further guidance on handling difficult ethnic diversity communication issues can be obtained from (26).

The challenge of working with colleagues

When a patient is deteriorating or nearing the end of their life differences of opinion among the multidisciplinary team can arise in terms of the patient's treatment or the treatment intent. Such differences can lead to difficult and strained working relationships.

Conflicts may occur when areas of expertise or roles overlap, leading to disagreements about the way forward with care. One example of this is when one colleague wishes to continue with an active treatment and another colleague following a clinical assessment believes the patient is dying and needs end of life care and wishes to implement the LCP. When these situations arise it is vital to attempt to discuss the situation with the person concerned. A framework for addressing such a situation is given in Box 5.6.

Box 5.6 Communicating with colleagues

Before a meeting:

◆ Warn your colleague you have something serious to discuss with them regarding a patient

◆ PAUSE to allow the information to sink in

◆ Negotiate a convenient time for a discussion on neutral territory if possible

At the meeting:

◆ Ensure that you are sitting at the same level as your colleague

◆ Introduce your self and role if necessary

◆ State the purpose of the meeting

◆ Outline your concerns briefly and allow time for information to be assimilated

◆ Invite the colleague to offer their perception of the situation

◆ Support their reasons and rationale

◆ State your own perception of the situation

◆ Try and negotiate a solution to help achieve the desired outcome

◆ Arrange a time to review the actions that have been agreed

Communicating effectively and sensitively with patients at the end of their lives and with their families can be one of the most difficult areas of care but in the words of Henri Nouven (1932–1996) 'The friend who can be silent with us in a moment of despair or confusion, who can stay with us in an hour of grief and bereavement, who can tolerate not knowing, not curing, not healing, and face us with the reality of our powerlessness, that is the friend who cares' (27) and in the philosophy of Confucius (28) when communicating:

◆ Think more

◆ Listen more

◆ Be cautious in your words and actions

◆ The advantage of doing things in this way is that you will have fewer regrets

In summary this chapter has outlined communication issues that commonly arise when implementing the LCP. Most of the techniques described are illustrated in two available CDs (29, 30). Another way in which health professionals can improve their communication skills is to raise their self-awareness of how they communicate by recording (with the patient's permission) an interaction with a patient and listening to themselves. It may be painful to do, but it has to be the responsibility of all working in end of life care as this will go a long way in ensuring that patients are receiving the best care possible, the ultimate aim of the LCP.

Further resources

Useful websites for communication skills training:

http://www.e-lfh.org.uk/projects/e-elca/index.html

http://www.endoflifecare.nhs.uk/eolc/

www.connected.nhs.uk

www.breakingbadnews.co.uk/index.asp

www.skillscascade.com/badnews.htm#

http://bmj.bmjjournals.com/cgi/content/full/321/7270/1233

www.newgrange-process.net

www.hospice-foundation.ie

References

1 King IM. (1971). *Towards a theory of nursing.* John Wiley and Sons Inc., New York.

2 Wilkinson SM. Factors which influence how nurses communicate with cancer patients. *J Adv Nurs.* 1991;**16**:677–88.

3 National Institute for Clinical Excellence (2004). *Guidance on cancer services: improving supportive and palliative care for adults with cancer.* The manual. http://www.nice.org.uk/nicemedia/pdf/csgspmanual.pdf (accessed 11 April 2008)

4 Department of Health (2007). *Cancer reform Strategy.* Crown Department of Health, London.

5 Department of Health (2000). *The NHS cancer plan.* Department of Health, London.

6 Healthcare Commission (2006). *The views of hospital patients in England.* Healthcare Commission, London.

7 White N (2009). In the interests of safety it is essential that doctors can communicate with their patients. Off the record Europe, bma.org.uk/bmanews (accessed 19 September 2009).

8 Wilkinson SM, Fellowes D, Leliopoulou C. Does truth-telling influence patients' psychological distress? *Europ J Palliat Care*, 2005;**12**(3):124–26.

9 Department of Health (2008). End of Life Strategy. Department of Health, London.

10 Bushkin E. Signposts of survivorship. *Oncol Nurs Forum*, 1995;**22**(3):537–43.

11 Macleod R (1991). *Patients with advanced breast cancer: the nature and disclosure of their concerns.* Unpublished MSc Thesis. University of Manchester, Manchester,UK.

12 Simpson M, Buckman R, Stewart M, Maguire P, Lipkin M, Novack D, et al. Doctor-patient communication: The Toronto consensus statement. *BMJ*, 1991;**303**:1385–7.

13 Taylor C, Graham J, Potts H, Candy J, Richards M, Ramirez AJ. Impact of hospital consultants' poor mental health on patient care. *Br J Psychiatry* 2007; **190**:268–69.

14 Fallowfield L, Jenkins V, Farewell V, Saul J, Duffy A, Eves R. Efficacy of a Cancer Research UK communication skills training model for oncologists: a randomised controlled trial. *Lancet*, 2002;**359**:650–56.

15 Fallowfield L, Jenkins V, Farewell V, Solis-Trapala I. Enduring impact of communication skills training: results of a 12-month follow-up. *Br J Cancer*, 2003;**89**:1445–49.

16 Wilkinson S, Linsell L, Perry R, Blanchard K. Effectiveness of a three-day communication skills course in changing nurses' communication skills with cancer/palliative care patients: A randomised controlled trial. *Palliat Med*, 2008;**22**:365–75.

17 Wilkinson S, Linsell L, Perry R, Blanchard K. Communication skills training for nurses working with patients with heart disease. *Brit J Cardiac Nurs*, 2008;**3**(10):476–81.

18 Wilkinson SM, Bailey K, Aldridge J, Roberts A. A longitudinal evaluation of a communication skills programme. *Palliat Med*, 1999;**13**:341–8.

19 Finset A, Ekeberg O, Eide H, Aspegren K. Long term benefits of communication skills training for cancer doctors. *Psycho-oncology*, 2003;**12**:686–93.

20 Thompson D. Too busy for assessment? *Nurs J*, 1990;**4**(21):35.

21 Quint JC (1967). *The nurse and the dying patient*. Macmillan, New York.

22 MCPCIL (2007). National Care of the Dying Audit Hospitals Generic Report Round 1 and (2009) ibid Round 2. www.mcpcil.org.uk

23 Silverman J, Kurtz S, Draper J (2005). *Skills for communicating with patients*, 2nd ed. Radcliffe Publishing, Oxford.

24 Gagan JM. Methodological notes on empathy. *Adv Nurs Sci*. 1983;**5**(2):65–72.

25 Koopmeiners L, Post-White J, Gutknecht S, Ceronsky C, Nickelson K, Drew D, et al. How healthcare professionals contribute to hope in patients with cancer. *Oncol Nurs Forum*, 1997;**24**(9):1507–13.

26 Kai J (ed) (2005). *PROCEED: Professionals responding to ethnic diversity and cancer*, Cancer Research, London, UK.

27 Nouven H (1990). *The Road to Daybreak: A Spiritual Journey*. Image Books. New York, USA.

28 Dan Yu (2009). *Confucius from the heart: Ancient Wisdom for todays world*. Macmillan, London.

29 Wilkinson S and Roberts A (2006). Communication skills course for health professionals in cancer care. CD Rom addressing assessment, handling difficult question, collusion and anger available from drsusie@btinternet.com

30 British Heart Foundation (2008). Communication skills in heart disease: Training for healthcare professionals addressing consultation skills, handling difficult questions, end of life issues, and communicating with colleagues. DVD available from tengwalls@bhf.org.uk

Chapter 6

Spiritual/religious issues in care of the dying

Peter Speck

How can the Liverpool Care Pathway for the Dying Patient (LCP) influence religious and/or spiritual care?

The essential components of a care pathway are the provision of a means for evaluating outcomes of care, provision of an agreed plan of care to which several professionals may contribute, and the use of current research to establish good practice thereby ensuring that patients receive quality care, especially towards the end of their life. The LCP will provide an effective means of ensuring that this aspect of care for dying patients is effectively taken into account and the appropriate spiritual needs met before and following the death.

Is there a research base for spiritual care in palliative care?

Links between religious affiliation and practice and health outcomes, sense of well being, mental health, and coping ability have been established in the USA where the overt practice of religious belief is more prevalent than in the UK. Recent studies in the UK into the wider concept of belief are indicating that for 69–71% of patients admitted into acute health care a belief system is important to them and is more predictive of outcome from the illness than the more commonly used psychological measures (1). Studies currently underway indicate that while some people may have moved away from established organized religion they still have an underlying spirituality which is of importance especially in the course of life crises (2). These studies are in an ageing population but have relevance given that people often live longer with their disease and enter end of life care at a greater age.

Why a special focus on spiritual care?

Various NHS guidance letters and the codes of good practice for professional groups (such as the UKCC Code for Nursing) indicate recognition that this aspect of care is integral to treating patients as people. Spiritual care is widely recognized to be an essential component of specialist palliative care, provided by a multi-professional team, as defined by the National Council for Hospice and Specialist Palliative Care Services (3). The integration of the various components of an holistic approach includes the psychological and the spiritual (4) as reflected in the NICE guidance (5) and the End of Life Strategy (6).

The LCP does not involve an in-depth spiritual assessment, but it does require exploration to ensure adequate support is made available to patients and carers as required. The first National Hospital Audit Report on the LCP (7) shows that assessment was only achieved for 34% of patients and 53% of carers, with a variance across the sample of 26% for patients and 14% for carers. In many cases the needs were not recorded (40% patients and 33% carers). The assessment and provision of these needs therefore still seem perplexing to health care staff with much lip service being paid to this aspect of care, with not even overt religious need always being addressed. This may be a problem with communication skills, over-sensitivity to the issues, or a blindness to the relevance for patients and carers. There were slightly better results for the two 12-hourly assessments of spiritual well-being for patients (61% achieved, but 36% not recorded). The results for the achievement of goals 6.1 and 6.2 (spiritual care) were further reduced in the 2009 Audit Report (8). There was also an increase in the proportion 'not documented'. In the context of 'reflective practice' the reasons for the apparent avoidance of this aspect of care should be addressed, with some reference to the earlier work of Ross and others (9,10).

An additional factor could be that some of the assessment tools developed so far have been too lengthy to use and better suited to research than clinical practice. Others are too tightly within a religious framework in spite of being called a spiritual assessment tool and can miss the wider non-religious spiritual need. However, there remains a need to discuss and explore needs through simple exploratory questions as indicated later in this chapter.

In the light of the second round audit, Recommendation 7 of the Report reiterates the earlier recommendation from Round 1:

> Hospitals need to identify the reasons for the relatively poorer performers on goals that deal with patient insight . . . and spiritual assessment (for both patients and carers). All health care workers caring for dying patients and their relatives/carers should have access to appropriate ongoing training and education in care of the dying (8).

The remainder of this chapter is offered as background to inform such an educational programme.

What is spiritual care?

Spiritual may be described as relating to the vital life essence of an individual. We may not always be consciously aware of its presence or perceive it as an area of need. However, it can assume considerable importance when our physical existence is threatened by disease and death. The outward expression of this vital force or existential dimension will be shaped and influenced by life experience, culture, and other personal factors. It integrates the various aspects of the person and is seen in the quality of relationships. Spirituality will, therefore, be unique for each individual. It may be understood as more than simply a search for meaning, but a search for *existential* meaning within the particular experience or life event, usually with reference to a power other than the self. There may be a developing sense of 'otherness'. The existential dimension is often expressed in terms of questions such as 'Who am I?' 'Does my life have any meaning and purpose?' and 'Has this illness the power to destroy me?' We may not, however, wish to use the term 'God' to describe the power but may talk about natural or cosmic forces, a sense of the other, a power in the universe etc. which has the ability to enable us to transcend the 'here and now' and sustain hope. We may not, therefore, always choose to express this spirituality through a religious framework.

Spiritual

A search for existential meaning within a life experience, usually with reference to a power other than the self, not necessarily called 'God', which enables transcendence and hope.

In essence we are talking about ways in which people in times of crisis or other formative moments in their life may become aware of a desire to understand or (existentially) make sense of what they are experiencing.

What is religious care?

A religion may be understood as a system of faith and worship which expresses an underlying spirituality.

This faith is frequently interpreted in terms of particular rules, regulations, customs, and practices as well as the belief content of the named religion. There is a clear acknowledgement of a power other than self, described as 'God' or 'enlightenment'. In some religious understandings this power is seen as an external controlling influence. In others the control is more from within the believer guiding and shaping behaviour. There is a long history of inter-relatedness between religion, healing, and medicine. When talking about religion one would not usually separate religion from spirituality, but neither should one use these terms interchangeably or assume that people who deny any religious affiliation have no spiritual needs. Some people will, therefore, have very clear religious views and needs arising out of their faith perspective. Others will not wish any religious ministry but may value appropriate companionship while exploring their spiritual questioning and needs.

Religion

A particular system of faith and worship expressive of an underlying spirituality and interpretive of what the named religion understands of 'God' or ultimate reality.

What about people who claim to be neither religious nor spiritual?

For some people the search for existential meaning will take a philosophical pathway and exclude any reference to a power other than themselves (e.g. existentialism/humanism/atheism). The individual, as a product of the individual's own personality and influence, will interpret and influence life events. Atheism, which is the denial of the existence of God, should be distinguished from agnosticism, which allows for a degree of uncertainty as to whether or not a deity exists. Some philosophical people will also claim to be spiritual and to have an appreciation of aesthetic experiences, but would not wish to embrace any notion of an external power that might be influential.

Philosophical

The search for existential meaning excludes any reference to a power other than from the self. Life events and the destiny of the individual being seen as manifestations of the individual's own personality as expressed individually and corporately.

A wider understanding of the word spiritual, as relating to the search for existential meaning within any given life experience, with the power to transcend that experience, allows us to consider spiritual needs and issues in the absence of any clear practice of a religion or faith. But this does not mean that they are to be seen as totally separated from each other (11). Rather they are inter-related. At its simplest level it is about affirming and respecting the humanity and personhood of the other person. This becomes important when trying to assess 'spiritual' need since health care staff may, incorrectly, deduce that those who decline anything religious have no spiritual needs.

When should we make the assessment?

This care pathway relates to the terminal or dying phase of a person's life and frequently this is not an opportune time to be asking detailed questions, or holding deep philosophical conversations. There should, however, be a simple screening on admission to ascertain any particular faith adherence and wish for referral to health care chaplain or faith leader should a crisis arise.

Ideally, assessment should be made and reviewed at various points in the illness. At each critical point in the person's life existential questions will arise and will be broached if the patient feels there are people around who will listen, and not leave them feeling 'silly' or morbidly negative.

It is good practice, therefore, for health care staff to have developed a reasonable understanding of the nature of their spiritual/pastoral support needs, their wishes for any (or no) specific religious support or ritual prior to and after death. Clearly needs change and in keeping with good practice in palliative care there should be regular re-assessment of all needs over time.

Some people will be very clear and articulate as to their needs while others may become frightened and panicky as they realize their life is drawing to a close. Late referrals to palliative care or chaplaincy may result in little opportunity to undertake a detailed assessment of any spiritual needs. If the patient expresses a wish to receive support or help in overcoming any fears or anxieties regarding their future, in terms of the illness or dying, it is important to respond appropriately. This might entail a more formal religious response of prayer, ritual (sacramental or otherwise), offering reassurance, or enabling the individual to express sorrow or sadness for past hurts or misdemeanours. It might also include sitting quietly with the person as they die and, if the care giver has a spiritual belief, praying for the dying person and family within one's own heart and mind. Any assessment of terminal agitation or pain should include consideration of other factors which could be exacerbating the pain in keeping with the model of 'total pain' (12). It may be too late for the individual to sort out all of the 'unfinished' business in their life. However, they can still benefit from experiencing affirming, accepting care from others whatever their belief system may be.

How can we assess this aspect of people's lives?

Much assessment to date has been of overt religious need with questions about religious affiliation and practice trailing off into silence or confusion if the answers are negative. Clearly there has to be a proper assessment of religious need but there also should be a way of reaching an understanding of what would be helpful for those who are not religious. This should not be an interrogation but more a conversation with a focus that allows key themes to be explored.

Suggested themes (using one's own phraseology) for exploratory questions might be:

- In the course of your life, with all its ups and downs, have you developed ways of making sense of the things that have happened to you?
- When life has been difficult what has helped you cope?

This may highlight the importance of the patient's family, philosophy of life ('I live one day at a time'), or belief system (religious, spiritual, or philosophical) as well as something of their current mental state. Hence it is not pushing people down a narrow religious pathway.

- Would you like to talk to someone about the effect your illness is having on you or your family?

This does not have to be a religious/faith leader, but when appropriate such a person should be introduced sensitively to patient and family to avoid the stereotypical image of the prelude to death.

If the conversation indicates that 'belief' is important then staff should enquire what form that belief takes and whether or not it is religious. (In our multi-cultural society we should perhaps now be talking of Faith Group and Faith Leaders and the sect/denomination of that faith group.)

Strict adherents of a particular faith group may well wish to have opportunity, either privately or with others, to continue to practice that faith. They may also, with their family, have both cultural and faith needs prior to and following their death. The wishes of the family and of the patient may be different and care is needed not to impose onto the patient the family's need. Thus the lapsed Catholic, or Jewish patient, has the priest or rabbi 'sent in' by the family, even though he/she does not wish to see them, and much distress may result.

Each faith tradition has its own rituals and religious practices that can support individuals and enable them to retain and/or strengthen their sense of connectedness with a 'higher power' or God. These religious needs may range from reading passages from the scripture or sacred writings of their faith, to the performance of specific religious rituals such as anointing with oil (see Box 6.1).

Box 6.1 Some religious needs

Prayer and reading of sacred writings

Privately or corporately: prayer time/meditation may require privacy

Availability of primary texts of the faith tradition

Commentary and instructive books concerning the faith

Religious rituals

Initiation rites, e.g. Christian baptism/circumcision

Holy Communion—specifically Christian

Ministry of healing—laying on of hands, anointing with oil

Acts of reconciliation—including healing of past hurts and forgiveness

Marriage—either religious ceremony or blessing after civil ceremony

Corporate acts of worship

- regular, especially on the 'holy' day

- at the time of festivals

- funeral/memorial services

Rites of passage around the time of death

What about the needs of different religious/faith groups

Palliative care workers should be aware of the importance of a multi-faith approach, consulting with the individual to avoid offering care in a stereotypical way. Cultural sensitivity is also important (13). Not all adherents of a faith group are equally strict and guidelines are no substitute for asking and exploring need with the patient or family. In all cases the family may wish to assist in the performance of Last Offices and may, therefore, appreciate the opportunity to do so.

Atheists or 'none'

1. If a patient puts 'none' against religion when coming into a Health Care setting it does not always mean that they have no religious faith. Sometimes it means that they do not wish to be contacted by a chaplain, or asked to make any religious commitment.

2. By creating a sensitive environment in which dying patients can express their feelings and fears, staff can fill an important pastoral role for patients of no stated religion.

3. However, it is important to understand that a chaplain's ministry has many dimensions. One essential element being to build a relationship of trust, understanding, and respect. This must take account of the patient's individual expectations, beliefs, and cultural patterns of behaviour, particularly in times of sickness and death, and make no attempt to impose particular religious views.

4. A sharing of this element of a chaplain's ministry and a gentle introduction of a visiting chaplain, if seen to be appropriate, may do much to comfort the dying patient and bereaved family.

Baha'i

1. The Baha'i faith is an independent world religion with its own laws and ordinances. Baha'is have a great respect for physicians and will wish to consult the best possible medical advice when they are ill.

2. Members are required to say an obligatory prayer each day and read from the scriptures of faith each morning and evening. This practice may continue when a Baha'i is dying and should be respected, as should the family or friends need to pray with the dying person.

3. Baha'is have a great respect for life, believing that their soul progresses after death.

4. There are no ritual procedures for the last offices and unless directed otherwise the usual procedure for the last offices can be carried out. Some families, especially those from an Iranian background, may wish to be present at the washing of the body. This should be respected where possible.

5. There is no objection in the Baha'i faith to post-mortem. Baha'is are taught to respect the body after death. There is also nothing in their teachings against organ donation.

6. Baha'i law forbids cremation, and states that the body should be buried at a site within one hours journey from the place of death. Baha'is are therefore encouraged to include a clause in their will stating their preference for burial.

Buddhist

There are several branches of Buddhism. It is advisable to ask the patient or the family about the nature of any observances to be made.

1. Buddhism stresses the need for the mind to be 'in touch' with the present moment. Buddhists may, therefore, be distressed if offered drugs which

impair consciousness, since great importance is often placed on the conscious state of mind at the time of death. Such medication may be refused.

2. A Buddhist patient may wish to practice 'private meditation' as death approaches. This should be respected where possible.

3. The family will advise on any procedures to be followed, in particular, if a Buddhist monk or sister should be contacted.

4. Where there are no known relatives or at the patient's request, contact can be made with a member of the Buddhist community. Some wards may have a list of names and telephone numbers available.

5. There are no ritual procedures for the last offices. Unless directed otherwise by the family, the usual procedure for the last offices can be carried out.

6. There is normally no objection to post-mortems.

7. By preference, it is usual for Buddhists to be cremated.

The Chinese community

Please discuss the needs of the patient and the family with the individuals concerned.

China has been a communist country for 40 years now, and the government has controlled and discouraged any following of religion. However, within China there are practising Buddhists, Christians, Muslims and many other faiths. For over two thousand years the teachings of Confucius have guided and shaped the Chinese government and how Chinese families lived. The worship of ancestors became a very important part of Chinese life, and it was felt that if respect was shown to elders and ancestors they would receive their blessings. Many Chinese people combine teachings, gods, and beliefs from the three main religions of ancient China: Confucianism, Taoism and Buddhism. Because of the wide variety of practice and belief it is important to discuss needs with the patient and family.

The Christian faith

The Christian faith is expressed through various denominations which have developed from differences of nationality, historical tradition, temperament, and belief. Individual expectations often vary, not only between the different denominations, but also within them. There are three main Christian denominational groupings in this country with at least one chaplain assigned to each grouping in most health care settings (Church of England/Anglican, Roman Catholic, and Free Church). The common ground between Christian denominations is considerable and enables health care chaplains to work as a team, while recognizing that people's needs may vary according to their Christian tradition. Special notice should be taken of two of the main sacraments of the Christian Church, Holy Communion and Baptism. Both of these sacraments are available to the patients through a chaplaincy or spiritual care team. An individual's own minister or parish priest may also offer pastoral care.

The need to be spiritually prepared for death can be of great importance, often unspoken, to those who may no longer attend formal worship in church.

The chaplain's ministry also extends to caring for the patient's relatives, and staff, particularly in times of obvious distress or sudden death, when the presence of the chaplain can bring comfort and support to the grieving family.

Anglican and Free Church patients

1. Assurance of spiritual security is vitally important to Christians facing death. A practicing Anglican or Free Church patient therefore will derive spiritual support and comfort from the presence of a chaplain as death approaches. The chaplain can offer the patient Holy Communion and appropriate prayers, or may simply sit with the patient and relatives to provide spiritual support and comfort.

2. Anglicans have no religious objections to post-mortems, and will decide for themselves in relation to post-mortems not required by law.

3. There are no religious preferences for burial or cremation; it is a matter of individual choice. However, respect for the body of the deceased is expected from all involved with any procedures following death.

4. It is very important in cases where unbaptized children are seriously ill or near to death that the parents are offered an opportunity to request baptism for their child. The priest should always be contacted in such cases although a lay person may baptize with water in the name of the Trinity, in the absence of a priest. This applies to all Christians, but some Free Church members who do not sanction infant baptism may wish their child to be named and blessed instead.

5. Broadly speaking, the Free Church chaplains are responsible for caring for the spiritual needs of those Christians who are not Roman Catholic or Church of England, and their ministry covers a wide range of members (14).

Roman Catholic patients

1. Roman Catholic patients will expect a visit from the priest who may bring Holy Communion and administer the Sacrament of the Sick (Anointing)

to those patients who request it. The Anointing is for all those who are suffering from a serious illness, disability, or old age.

2. When a Roman Catholic patient is near to death the priest will also, if possible, give them the Last Rites (Viaticum). This consists of the patient receiving Holy Communion for the last time (Viaticum means 'Bread for the journey'). Once a patient has died, the family may wish the priest to lead the Prayers for the Dead as a last mark of respect and as a support to those who grieve. If in doubt, a priest should always be called, because when a patient states his/her religion to be Roman Catholic, this is what they would usually expect.

Hindu

Hindu beliefs and practices vary considerably. Where at all possible it is advisable to ask the patient or the family about the nature of the particular observances to be carried out.

Most Hindus require time for meditation and prayer, and this will be most evident in terminal illness, when small idols or pictures of gods may be kept under the pillow, or by the bed, as may praying beads and flowers or charms. Recognition should be given to the support, comfort, and help which Hindus derive from these traditions.

Hindu priests very often wish to perform the last rites, but in their absence it would give comfort to the Hindu patient to have some verses from the Bhagavad Gita read to them, if they so desire.

A Hindu priest may be contacted via the family themselves.

1. After the death of the patient, surgical attachments must be removed, care must be taken *not to remove any threads* which have been put around the neck or wrist by the priest.

2. The body is then left for the family's arrival as they may wish to perform the last offices. It is permissible for the nursing staff to straighten the limbs, close the eyes.

3. As there is usually no restriction on non-Hindus handling the body, and no ritual washing of the body, it is permissible for nursing staff, in consultation with the family, to perform the last offices.

4. In circumstances where the family wishes to perform the last offices, staff should respect this practice and sensitively offer the family assistance.

5. The body should then be wrapped in a plain *white* sheet and placed in the mortuary. It is acceptable, once the death certificate has been provided, for the relatives to take the deceased home.

6. It is Hindu practice that grief is expressed openly with physical gestures, hands being held and people embracing, much physical comfort being derived from this practice. Staff should provide a quiet place, away from other patients, where the relatives can grieve in this way for an acceptable period of time.

7. Although there are no rules about post-mortems, relatives will often consider them extremely objectionable and disrespectful to the dead. This issue should be handled with great sensitivity when advising Hindu relatives of the need for a post-mortem, e.g. by order of the coroner.

8. It is normal for Hindus to be cremated after death. Children under five years of age, however, are always buried, never cremated. Staff should be aware of this practice to avoid causing offence or distress to the family.

Jehovah's Witnesses

1. Jehovah's Witnesses have a high regard for the medical profession and are appreciative of the care and dedication shown to them by health care staff. They are quite willing to accept medical treatment with the exception of *blood transfusions* or *blood derivatives*. This stand is based on the command given in the Bible to abstain from taking blood into the body as the life of the donor is within the blood (Leviticus 17:14 and Acts 15:20–29). Recent statements indicate that the receipt of blood/blood products in a serious life threatening event may not always lead to automatic expulsion from the Kingdom Hall. However, this should still be treated with sensitivity.

2. The seriously ill or dying Jehovah's Witness has no morbid fear of death; it is looked upon as a sleep-like condition from which there will eventually be a resurrection as specifically stated in God's word. (John 11:25).

3. The situation may arise where the patient is the only Jehovah's Witness in a family. Care must be taken to handle this situation with the family sensitively if the patient's Presiding Overseer has, *at the patient's request*, been informed.

4. Jehovah's Witnesses do not have any 'last rites' service or similar ministry.

5. It is therefore acceptable for last offices procedure to be followed.

6. There is no particular preference for cremation or burial, it is entirely a matter of individual choice. Jehovah's Witnesses do not usually object to post-mortems.

7. In certain cases, Jehovah's Witnesses nearing death may indicate the wish to donate organs for transplantation. Before taking such a decision,

Jehovah's Witnesses would wish for a quiet place to prayerfully consider the matter before making a personal conscientious decision. Staff should be considerate of this and provide a quiet place for them to do this.

Jewish patients

As Jewish beliefs and rites vary considerably with the branch of Judaism to which the person belongs, the wishes of the family should be sought regarding any particular observances to be made.

1. If a Jewish patient is dying, the next of kin should be informed, and if it is the wish of the patient and/or relatives contact should be made with the patient's own Rabbi or synagogue. Similarly upon the death of a Jewish patient this procedure should be followed. The Rabbi will decide the appropriate form of response.

2. Traditionally the body of the deceased should remain as it was when the death occurred. The body should remain untouched for 30 minutes, during which time surgical attachments should remain in place.

3. Once this period of time has elapsed, if the relatives have not arrived, or it has not been possible to obtain the services of a Jewish chaplain, it is permissible for the nursing staff (*wearing disposable gloves*) to carry out the following procedure:

   (a) The *clothes should not be removed*.

   (b) The eyes and mouth should be closed.

   (c) The fingers of each hand should be straightened and the hands and arms should be placed parallel to the body. Similarly, the legs and feet should be straightened.

   (d) Any tubes or artificial limbs should be removed and any incisions plugged so as to prevent or stem a flow of blood or body fluids.

   (e) Any *excess* dirt should be wiped away and washed off, but the body should not otherwise be washed.

   (f) The body *still fully clothed* should be wrapped in the bottom sheet. To enable the mortuary technician to respect Jewish tradition, it would be helpful if the body of the deceased could be labelled 'Jewish'.

4. Jewish law requires the body to remain totally intact after death and regards the carrying out of a post-mortem as a desecration of the body. Care should therefore be taken to ensure that the relatives of Jewish patients are not

asked to consent to a post-mortem unless required by law, as this is likely to cause offence and distress.

5. Occasionally, a request may be made by members of the family or Jewish community to remain with the deceased either at the bedside or after the body has been removed to the mortuary. (A professional 'watcher' may be used). This request is in keeping with Jewish tradition and should be treated with respect.

6. Jewish law insists on the funeral taking place as soon as possible after death, usually within 24 hours. It is therefore important that a death certificate is made available at the earliest possible opportunity, enabling arrangements to commence.

7. Deaths usually have to be registered in the Borough in which they occur. No provision is made by the Registrar within many areas for the registering of deaths on Saturdays, Sundays, and Bank Holidays.

8. While cremation may be more acceptable to some Reformed Jews it is better not to make a reference to cremation unless a relative raises the issue. Burial in a Jewish cemetery is the only option for Orthodox Jews.

9. All still-born babies should be buried and, in the event of a miscarriage, the parents should be consulted about the disposal of the foetus to enable them to consult their Rabbi for guidance.

10. In the event of a pregnant woman dying without there being any possibility of safely delivering the child, the mother and child should be buried together without Caesarean section being performed.

11. It can be a source of considerable comfort to a Jew to know that the staff can say a prayer with them if no immediate family is available.

Mormon

Properly known as 'The Church of Jesus Christ of Latter-Day Saints'

1. Mormons who have undergone a special Temple Ceremony wear a sacred undergarment. This intensely private item is normally worn at all times. It may be removed for laundering or surgical operations but at all times must be considered as *private* and treated with respect.

2. There are no religious objections to blood transfusion.

Diet

Mormons are very health conscious. They are not normally vegetarians, but will only eat meat very sparingly, avoiding products which contain quantities of blood.

They are concerned about stimulants, therefore do not drink tea or coffee. The availability of milk and fruit juices will be appreciated. Alcohol and tobacco are forbidden.

Care for the Dying

1. There are no ritual acts for the dying

2. Contact with other members of the church is important

3. 'Home teachers' will visit and support church members

4. At death, if the sacred garment is worn it must be replaced on the body once last offices are completed

5. Burial is preferred

6. A Bishop from the local Mormon Church will be available to give blessings and minister to the sick. The Bishop will offer solace and help with funeral arrangements

7. Mormons have no religious objections to post-mortem examination or organ donation.

Muslim

It is not always necessary to call an Imam when a Muslim is dying as the family will traditionally stay with the patient to pray. However, if the family are not present, and/or if the patient requests it, contact may be made with an Imam at the local mosque. Muslim beliefs and practices may vary considerably. Where possible it is advisable to ask the family the nature of any observances to be made.

1. Following the death of a Muslim, the body should remain untouched for 30 minutes; surgical attachments etc should remain in place.

2. There is usually no objection to non-Muslims handling the body, provided they *wear disposable gloves*. The family may like to perform the last offices themselves and should be consulted in this matter where possible.

3. With the family's approval it is permissible for nursing staff to carry out the following procedure:

   (a) Close the eyes and the mouth.

   (b) The fingers of each hand should be straightened and the hands and arms should be placed parallel to the body. Similarly, the legs and feet should be straightened.

   (c) Any tubes or artificial limbs should be removed and any incisions plugged so as to prevent a stem or a flow of blood or body fluids.

(d) Any *excess* dirt should be *wiped* off.

(e) The head should be turned towards the right shoulder, which will enable the body to be buried facing Mecca.

(f) The body should be wrapped, *unwashed* and still clothed, in a plain white sheet and placed in the mortuary. It is helpful to denote that the patient is a Muslim on the relevant documentation.

4. Muslim tradition necessitates the washing of the body to be carried out by Muslims of the same sex. This will take place either at the family home or sometimes at the mosque.

5. Muslim law insists on the carrying out of a funeral as soon as possible after death, usually within 24 hours. It is important, therefore, that a death certificate be available at the earliest possible opportunity to enable these arrangements to be made.

6. Post-mortems are not usually allowed except by order of the coroner. In other circumstances the next of kin may wish to consult the Islamic authorities before making a decision.

7. Grief may be displayed openly. Staff should endeavour to provide a quiet place for the weeping relatives to grieve for an acceptable period of time, away from patient areas.

8. Muslims are always buried, *never* cremated.

Pagan

The title 'Pagan' does not describe a uniform group but is descriptive of a variety of traditions which have their origins in ancient rituals which are claimed to be more in tune with the elemental forces of the universe. There are many forms of paganism in the UK but the importance of a right relationship with elemental forces is integral to the rituals as well as the health and well being of the devotee, be they a Druid, a White Wicca, or an adherent of another pagan group. Most members will inform staff of any particular needs.

Sikh

1. If a Sikh patient is dying, the family will wish to be informed at the earliest possible opportunity to enable the following traditions to be followed:

(a) The Priest or family will read hymns to the dying Sikh from the Holy Book—the Ad Granth.

(b) Before death occurs, a Sikh is given holy water by the Priest or family, a few drops being placed in the mouth. Holy water is obtainable from the Temple, or some families will have their own supply brought from the Golden Temple of Amritsar in India. A sensitive regard for this practice will bring comfort to the Sikh patient and the grieving relatives.

In the absence of any relatives, contact can be made with the local Sikh Community—the President of the Local Sikh Temple will be pleased to advise.

2. After the death of the patient, surgical attachments can be removed and if the family have not arrived it is permissible for the nursing staff to straighten the limbs, close the eyes and support the jaw. If the family are present, their permission should be sought before carrying out this procedure, as they may wish to do this themselves. Staff should respect this practice, and sensitively offer assistance where appropriate.

3. It is normal Sikh practice for the family to wash and dress the body, such practice usually being carried out at home. However, some Sikh families may wish to carry out this procedure in the place where the person has died. Staff should respect this, and sensitively offer assistance where appropriate.

4. If the family do not wish to carry out the last offices it is permissible for the nursing staff, in consultation with the family, to carry out the following procedure:

   (a) *Wipe* away any *excess* dirt. The body should *not* be washed, unless the family indicate otherwise.

   (b) Plug any incisions to prevent or stem the flow of blood or body fluids.

   (c) The turban worn by male Sikhs should be left in place, as should any small combs which may be in the hair.

   (d) The body should then be wrapped *unwashed* (unless the family have indicated otherwise) in a plain white sheet, and removed to the mortuary.

5. Sikhs are normally cremated, and tradition insists that this takes place as soon as possible. Families will be appreciative if the death certificate is available at the earliest possible opportunity.

6. It is usual for still-born babies to be buried, the parents undertaking all the funeral rites.

7. The subject of post-mortem should be treated with sensitivity when advising that this may be required by order of the coroner

What of the non-religious spiritual needs?

The assessment of spiritual need often relates to trying to assess the extent to which the sick person feels disconnected from those people or powers that enable the person to retain some sense of existential meaning and purpose in their life under more normal circumstances. The extent to which we are, or wish to be connected, will depend on previous life experience as well as the present situation or our prognosis for the future. The prospect of imminent or untimely death may well trigger off existential questions for people. The answers to these questions may or may not draw on a belief in a power other than self. There is much variety in the understanding of the nature of that power for those who do hold such a belief system, and it is often explored and understood in relationship. People who do not profess any form of religious faith may still wish to have opportunity to be quiet, to reflect, and to commune with whatever forces or powers they feel are beneficial to them. In the various ways in which palliative care is made available to people there needs to be opportunity to explore the impact of the illness and its consequences for both the quality of life and the ultimate quality of the death event. Spiritual well being may be a valuable resource to support people as they come to terms with terminal illness and try to retain this sense of identity in the face of illness and treatments which may threaten to fragment it. Failure to identify and sustain this resource may contribute to the experience of spiritual pain or distress.

Spiritual pain is linked to

+ A sense of hopelessness
+ Focus on suffering rather than pain
+ Feelings of guilt and/or shame
+ Unresolved anger
+ Inability to trust
+ Lack of inner peace
+ Sense of disconnectedness or fragmentation.

Spiritual pain is often identified in people whose physical/emotional pain fails to adequately respond to recognized approaches to symptom relief. It is often linked to issues relating to a sense of hopelessness or meaninglessness. It may be expressed as suffering (rather than 'pain') indicating that there seems no meaning or purpose to the pain and the experience is all-encompassing rather than localized or specific. Feelings of guilt or shame may be expressed and an inability to trust—other people, oneself, or 'God'. This can lead to disconnectedness from a previous religious or belief position, or from other people, which can result in greater <u>dis</u>-ease or lack of inner peace. While some of these things can be tackled from a psychosocial perspective, when they assume an ultimate or existential significance the intervention needs to be of a spiritual nature.

The setting in which palliative care is delivered will influence the range of available activities and resources. A home care team may have a more limited opportunity than a day care unit or an in-patient hospice unit. Providing specialist palliative care in a busy acute hospital ward may also restrict what it is possible to provide. It is significant that many of the complementary forms of therapy have a clear focus on the individual person and on trying to assist that individual in their search for what many describe as 'inner peace' and therefore related to spiritual need and development. Thus aromatherapy, head or foot massage, visualization or art therapy may all enable the person to explore and express aspects of themselves and their experience of illness and treatment in the hope of transcending some of the more difficult aspects. Reminiscence (written and spoken) and guided imagery are important aspects of care which may help with easing spiritual pain in terms of allowing some healing or reconciliation of the person with their past. Most patients wish to engage in activities which they believe address them more clearly as a person, or which nourish the non-material aspects of their life.

It must not be forgotten that there are also many patients who may not wish to be active but who still value having an aesthetically good setting. For such patients especially touch, smell, views through a window, and beauty can become very important. In this situation it is especially important to focus on the art of 'being with' rather than always wanting to be active and 'do to'.

Who should meet the needs assessed?

In many cases spiritual care will be the specific remit of properly appointed faith leaders. Currently these will usually be of a Christian tradition but new guidance on the appointment of health care chaplains has enabled Trusts and other health care providers to appoint spiritual care givers from non-Christian traditions where the numbers of patients justify this. Where this is not currently the case those appointed to provide spiritual care should establish links with other faith communities and try to obtain the services of people who can confidently offer supportive care and spiritual support to terminally ill people. The Christian concept of pastoral care is not understood in the same way by some faith groups. For example in Judaism and Islam the faith leader (Rabbi or Imam) would primarily be a teacher who would instruct what to read, what to eat or not eat, what rituals to follow around the time of death. However, the family or other designated community members would visit to support. In the case of Judaism many of these visitors, however, would studiously avoid talking about the imminent death and direct the individual to thoughts of the goodness of God, and blessings of this life. Interpreting the approaches of another culture and faith is fraught with difficulty and we need always to remember we speak from an ethnocentric context however well informed we may be (13). In all cases the patient should be our guide in terms of needs and of who should meet them.

In many cases spiritual care will be provided by the very staff who have assessed the needs since the patient has developed a relationship of trust with that individual. The role of the official pastoral care givers may well be to support the staff as they follow through with the patient, rather than taking over. Where very specific rituals are required then faith leader and staff could also work together and complement each other's role.

In many faith traditions the family will be the key providers of spiritual support and will often initiate prayers, specific rituals, or requests for more informed ministry. It is always good practice to consult with the family as to what their wishes may be and this should be a clear component of the LCP.

Acknowledgement

I wish to acknowledge the contribution of Sister Ursula Reynolds Director of Pastoral Care at the Marie Curie Centre, Liverpool, for background research into the religious needs of many of the major faith communities within the UK.

References

1 King M, Speck P, Thomas A. The effect of spiritual beliefs on outcome from illness. *Social Science and Medicine* 1999;**48**:1291–99

2 Speck P, Bennett K, Coleman PG, Mills M, McKiernan F et al (2005). Elderly bereaved spouses: Issues of belief, well-being and support. In Walker A *Growing Older: Understanding Quality of Life in Old Age*. Maidenhead, Open University Press.

3 NCHS www.hospice-spc-council.org.uk

4 World Health Organisation. (1990). *Technical Report Series*, 804. W.H.O. Geneva.

5 National Institute for Health and Clinical Excellence (2004) *Improving Supportive and Palliative Care for Adults with Cancer*. NICE, London.

6 Department of Health (2008) *The End of Life Care Strategy*. DH, London.

7 MCPCIL (2007) National Care of the Dying Audit Hospitals Generic Report Round 1 and (2009) ibid Round 2. www.mcpcil.org.uk

8 MCPCIL (2009) National Care of the Dying Audit Hospitals Generic Report Round 2. www.mcpcil.org.uk

9 Ross LA (1997) *Nurses' Perceptions of Spiritual Care*. Avebury, Aldershot.

10 Dein S. The role of health professionals in spiritual care: attitudes, practices and interventions. *Eur J Palliat Care*. 2009;16(6):296–300.

11 Speck P (1988). *Being There: pastoral care in time of illness*. SPCK, London.

12 Saunders C. (1967). *The Management of Terminal Illness*. Arnold, London.

13 Speck P (2001). Cultural issues. In *Palliative care for non-cancer patients* (eds. J.M. Addington-Hall and I.J.Higginson). Oxford University Press, Oxford.

14 Speck P A full list of recognized 'Free Churches' is obtainable from: The Free Church Federal Council, Tavistock Square, London.

Chapter 7

Supporting family and friends as death approaches and afterwards

Carole Mula

The focus of this chapter is care after death, section 3 of the Liverpool Care Pathway (LCP), and is designed to guide health professionals to care for family and friends as the death of a loved one approaches and to provide support immediately after the death which can impact positively on the family's experience of loss (1).

The importance of appropriately assessing, addressing, and reviewing the needs of families and friends both during a patient's life and into bereavement in order to be able to offer a support system to help the family cope during the patient's illness and in their own bereavement has been recommended in recent reports (2–5).

Bereavement

The loss of a close family member often engenders powerful and sometimes unfamiliar feelings and thoughts and is recognized to be one of the most traumatic types of bereavement (6). Furthermore, associated physical and mental health consequences of bereavement are well documented (7) as is an increase in the mortality rate of bereaved persons (8).

The terms bereavement, grief, and mourning are often used interchangeably. However, there are very important distinctions between them based on the way loss is understood. For the purpose of this chapter the following definitions will be used:

- Bereavement is understood to refer to the objective situation of having lost someone significant
- Grief is the reaction to bereavement, defined as a primarily emotional (affective) reaction to the loss of a loved one through death
- Mourning is the social expressions or acts expressive of grief that are shaped by the practices of a given society or cultural group (9).

A key aim of bereavement support is to minimize associated health risks by offering proactive support to those most vulnerable. However, it is important to recognize that the majority of bereaved people do not need 'outside' help or sophisticated support to cope with their grief. They are likely to handle their bereavement with nothing more than information, guidance, and reassurance about the normality of their grief and associated feelings. They manage their grieving with emotional support from their family, friends, and social networks together with their own internal resources (10). Only a minority of people, primarily those who are left feeling overwhelmed and insecure, particularly if they have pre-existing social and psychological vulnerabilities are at risk of experiencing persistent physical and mental problems (11).

Optimum bereavement support is influenced by effective communication between relatives and health professionals. This requires professionals to tailor their communications to individual information needs. However, this assumes that health professionals are able to both cope with loss and discuss loss openly and sensitively. In reality, many professionals find death and dying difficult to discuss with both patients and families (12) as this may trigger personal experiences of loss and foreseeable future losses; or act as a reminder of one's own and others' mortality. Health professionals' fears and uneasiness around discussing and coping with death need to be addressed, to enable them to cope in supporting relatives' immediate grief reactions effectively. If these issues have not been addressed, professionals may adopt blocking tactics (see Chapter 5), that may result in the bereaved feeling abandoned, isolated, and unsupported.

'Making decisions about who may be vulnerable after bereavement is a complex process that relies on the nurse's knowledge of risk factors and having sufficient time and skills to work with family members' (13). Reviews of the extensive literature on risk factors conclude that differences in health outcomes are influenced by:

- Events and circumstances leading up to the death (e.g. sudden death)
- Meaning of the relationship with the deceased (e.g. unfinished business)
- Personal vulnerability of the bereaved person (e.g. newly divorced, experiencing other concurrent loss)
- Availability of social support and economic resources (10,11,13,14):

The vulnerability of the bereaved individual is increased by the number of risk factors present. The collective presence of risk factors can be used to decide the level of support needed pre-emptively (13,15) (Table 7.1).

Checklists are available to help professionals assess risks (16). However, evidence suggests that current risk assessment tools have limited reliability and

Table 7.1 Risk factors that may complicate bereavement (data adapted from Kissane 2008, Relf 2008)

Events and circumstances leading up to the death	Short or long history of illness Sudden or unexpected death Traumatic death Stigmatized (e.g. AIDS) Suicide Homicide No body has been found
Meaning of the relationship with the deceased	Overly close/dependant Ambivalent (e.g. hostility at infidelity, gambling, alcoholism) Unrecognized (e.g. an affair)
Personal vulnerability of the bereaved person	History of or current mental health illness, e.g. depression Low self-esteem Additional stresses and concurrent life events Multiple losses
Availability of social support and economic resources	Financial difficulties Isolation Poor family functioning Lack of social support

are inconsistently used in practice (17). More recently, it has been suggested that an integrated approach should be adopted that examines coping and incorporates measures of resilience in addition to risk factors (13,16). It is argued that individuals with better coping mechanisms are more resilient, and this influences their health outcomes rather than the presence of risk factors alone (18).

Anticipatory grief

The evidence related to assessment of individual grief reactions prior to death is limited. It has been reported that anticipatory grief (grieving prior to death) occurs, although what to do about it remains unclear (19,20). Anticipatory grief experiences were first identified by Lindemann (21) as early as 1944 and later described in more detail by Schoenberg et al. (22) as, the emotional experiences some people have before the loss of a loved one. It involves a complex range of cognitive, physical, and social responses made by the dying person, as well as the soon to be bereaved, prior to death. Grief experiences that take place before death are different in duration and form from those that take place after death. In anticipatory grieving the patient and their relatives are often experiencing similar emotions during a period of sustained uncertainty. It provides the grieving relative with the opportunity to grieve in advance of death, but can also complicate what people refer to as, 'the working through process', by the griever realizing their emotional feelings about and towards the dying person before death. Early evidence indicates that preparation for the loss can be a beneficial aspect of anticipatory grief. However, Rando (23) suggests that prolonged duration between diagnosis and death, especially in younger people, is associated with a greater likelihood of difficulties arising. Where the loss relates to older people, there are contradictions in bereavement outcomes; although in general, bereavement outcomes are considered more positive when a period of preparation allowed grieving to take place prior to death (24,25). It is therefore important to establish how the relatives are coping with caring for the person and their own anticipatory grief.

Current risk management strategies

Relf et al. (10) have developed a decision-making pathway to help professionals assess an individual's potential needs. It is separate from the LCP (and should not be confused). This decision-making pathway has primarily been developed for hospice care where professionals generally have the skills and resources to undertake in-depth assessments of relatives' needs. However, elements of the pathway may be transferrable across different healthcare settings.

This pathway focuses on the identification of an individual's coping responses, to establish those most vulnerable who are likely to need professional support. The support then offered, may vary according to individual need, from group or individual befriending through to bereavement counselling and therapy. This process requires dialogue with family members together with observation of their reactions that should start pre-bereavement and form part of the ongoing assessment (10). It is important to seek permission from relatives and friends to allow professionals to keep information about them in this way.

This pathway adopts the concept that grief reactions fall into two categories: overwhelming distress and/or a desire to retain control (26). It is suggested that the majority of people use both ways to manage their loss and may oscillate between overwhelming feelings of distress and maintaining control. This is dependent on personal resources and circumstantial factors surrounding the loss and it is these factors that affect an individual's resilience or vulnerability (see Tables 7.2 and 7.3) (26). Their grief reactions (Box 7.1) of overwhelming distress or control are not in themselves indicators of risk (Figure 7.1) (10).

Table 7.2 Personal resources

Difficulties in dealing with past stressors	More vulnerable
Physical or psychological existing stressors	
Adequate inner resources to meet demands of the loss	
Hopeful outlook	More resilience
Positive past experiences	

Adapted from Relf M, Machin L, Archer N (2008) with permission. © Help the Hospices

Table 7.3 Circumstantial factors

Difficult death	
Caring for elderly parents/children	More vulnerable
Relationship/financial/housing problems	
Events surrounding the death are positive	
Support available	More resilience
Manageable additional demands	

Adapted from Relf M, Machin L, Archer N (2008) with permission. © Help the Hospices

Box 7.1 Types of grief reactions

◆ Controlled: little or no emotional response to the situation, matter of fact in discussions about the illness and its outcome, does not seek support for themselves, self-reliant, difficultly in responding to other people's emotions, major focus on practical concerns

◆ Overwhelmed: tearful, anxious, agitated, fearful, pessimistic, depleted resources, lack of trust in themselves, frequently seeking reassurance, unable to process information, demanding of staff attention, critical of patient's treatment

◆ Resilient: shows emotion but distress is not persistent, able to describe situations coherently, able to engage in discussions about the illness and its outcome, open to the changing needs and emotions of the patient, accepting of help and support, can take 'time out'

◆ Vulnerable: avoids facing impending loss, does not demonstrate coping mechanisms, does not feel hopeful that strength and meaning may come from the experience, angry, depressed, difficulty in relating to staff, unpredictable responses to discussions about the illness and its outcome, ambivalent about accepting support.

Adapted from Relf M, Machin L, Archer N (2008) with permission. © Help the Hospices

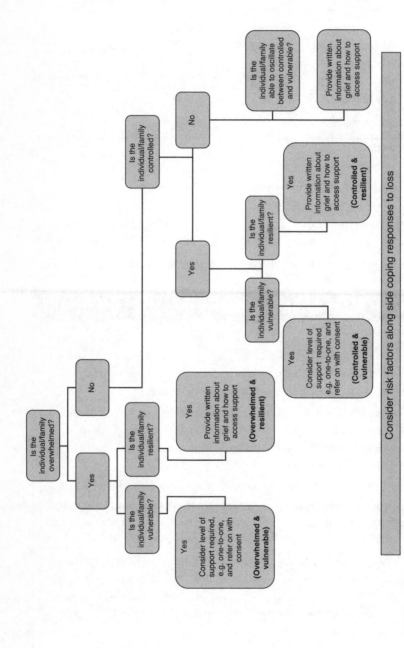

Fig. 7.1 Flow chart of the decision making pathway for bereavement needs assessment.

Key considerations alongside risk factors

In summary, people dealing with other stressful life demands whose personal capacity is reduced and circumstantial risk heightened, are more likely to experience a significant impact when death occurs. They are also likely to experience more persistent feelings or loss of control. These mourners are more likely to need formal bereavement support.

What is involved in making an assessment?

Guidance on the areas to be addressed when undertaking a needs assessment are highlighted in Table 7.4; and Figure 7.1 illustrates a flow chart to guide the assessment process.

Social and cultural considerations

Consideration must be given to the social and cultural background of the bereaved individual as this can influence their reaction to loss and their level of resilience and vulnerability. A fundamental variation across all cultures and social circumstances is the private versus public experience of mourning. In some cultures, mourning is a social affair whereas in others, such as the UK, it is a private controlled affair (27) where expression of feelings can be inhibited by the perceived need for emotional control. In anticipation of those cultures where mourning is a social and expressive affair, it may be preferable to provide a secluded area for the people concerned.

Involvement of social and pastoral workers is important, as they have an important role in preparing families for the death of a patient (28). (See Chapter 6.)

Table 7.4 Managing the needs assessment

- Gather information through observation and discussion with relatives
- Formal and informal discussions by the multi-professional team to develop a more robust understanding of individual ways of coping
- Document assessment through use of an assessment form. This documentation is best begun *pre-bereavement* but should be completed as soon as possible after the patient's death
- Make decisions about the type and level of follow-up to be offered
- Administer the process to ensure that all families are included
- Proactively offer services to those considered to be vulnerable and document the appropriate support
- Give written information about grief and how to access support to all bereaved families including those who are not considered to be vulnerable.

Adapted from Relf M, Machin L, Archer N (2008) with permission. © Help the Hospices

Social workers have experience of working with populations from varying cultures, ages, socioeconomic status, and non-traditional families and can provide additional support, advice, and care for families facing death, grief, and bereavement. Pastoral workers and religious advisors will, in many cases, help to ascertain the patient's wishes; make any necessary cultural practices clear before death (29); and provide support immediately after the death for the family.

Bereavement can be a particularly stressful time for families who are unable to adequately speak the native language of the country where the deceased has died. They may have difficulties in expressing themselves and making their wishes understood. In such cases the services of an interpreter would be appropriate.

Preparing the family for the imminent death

For many relatives, being present at the time of death is very important. Thus, once a patient deteriorates and death is imminent, the family should be gently informed of the changes. Euphemisms should not be used as these can be misinterpreted by the family (see Chapter 5). If the family are not present, the named person previously identified on the LCP should be contacted and informed of the change in condition, allowing them the opportunity of being with the patient if they so wish. Support and availability of staff for the family is crucial. The family need the opportunity to voice their concerns and ask any questions. It is helpful to listen and acknowledge these sensitively and give appropriate information on the next possible stages. However, few people are ever prepared for the death of a loved one and even when the patient is lingering, the death can still appear sudden and come as a shock (29). To prepare them for the next stages it is helpful to use words such as the patient's 'pulse is getting weaker' or 'I can hardly feel a pulse'.

Although the family may be with the patient at the time of death, some may not be aware that death has actually occurred. In such circumstances, the family need to be informed with empathy that the patient has died. The word 'died' should always be used rather than euphemisms such as 'passed away', 'passed on', as these reinforce the taboo surrounding death and dying that exists in some societies.

If the relatives were not present at the time of death, they should be contacted as previously agreed. This can pose challenges for professionals as to whether this news should be given over the phone or whether telling a beneficent lie such as, the patient 'has taken a turn for the worse and they should come in immediately' is preferable. Kent and McDowell's (30) literature review of bereavement in acute care settings, suggests that whenever possible relatives should not be informed by phone of the death unless they have far to travel.

However, the way in which death is communicated is more important than whether this is carried out over the telephone or face-to-face.

Last offices

Goal 10 of the LCP focuses on last offices and treating the deceased with respect and dignity. Often nurses care for the deceased immediately after death. In some environments such as care homes, hospitals, and hospices, care workers are also involved in this care. They manage the transition between a person's body being considered as alive to being dead through the process of last offices (31), sometimes referred to as 'laying out'. Last offices centre on preparing the deceased to ensure a physical appearance that is in keeping, as best as possible, with how the patient looked when they were alive. Family members may wish to be involved in the process of last offices and nurses should offer them the opportunity to do so.

For many families, spending time with the body of a loved one will be an important stage in the bereavement process and can help to facilitate the grief process by providing an opportunity to say goodbye (30,32).

It is important that nurses are able to demonstrate competence and reverence in caring for the deceased patient, carrying out the procedure both quietly and professionally. This in turn reflects positively on the care that has been provided for the patient. Relatives will be supported by knowing that the patient has been treated with respect. An important part of the administrative process at the time of death is identifying the relatives' wishes in relation to the deceased's possessions. These must be dealt with according to the organization's policy. The appearance of the deceased and how personal belongings are handled can transform the experience for families (1).

Nurses must also adhere to local policy and procedures for the ritual of last offices, infection risk, and management of invasive equipment such as indwelling urinary catheters and subcutaneous lines.

The key points in performing last offices, are shown in Box 7.2 .It is vital that nurses do not impose their own faith or traditional practices on the deceased or their relatives and respect their spiritual, religious, and cultural needs.

Organ/tissue donation

A further consideration at the time of or near death is that of organ or tissue donation as prompted by Goal 11. This can be a difficult subject to initiate. It is important to establish whether this has been considered either by the family or the deceased in the past. There is little evidence that organ donation or

Box 7.2 Last offices: key points

Nurses must:

- Show respect and dignity to the deceased
- Ensure the deceased appears well groomed and presentable
- Be respectful when managing the deceased's personal property
- Complete clear and timely documentation
- Communicate openly and honestly with the bereaved relatives
- Care for the deceased and their relatives in line with local and national guidelines and policies
- Consider cultural rites and respect diversity

refusal has any significant impact on the grieving process over the long term (33). Some organizations have transplant or bereavement coordinators who are responsible for the care of the person who has died, speaking to the relatives, facilitating the donation procedure, and providing support to the relatives before, during, and after donation. Patients, who die supported by the LCP, may be eligible to donate organs and tissue. Tissue donation can be donated up to 24 hours after the heart has stopped beating; the most common donations being the eye, bone, skin, heart valves, tendon, and cartilage. Each case is examined individually as variances occur, depending on the specific case, such as diagnosis and past medical history (34,35). The guidelines for organ and tissue donation vary across countries and thus it is imperative to follow local guidance.

Medical and legal issues

Legal requirements regarding verification and certification of death must be complied with.

While it may be clear that the patient has died, the death must be verified as soon as possible by an appropriate health professional, (usually the doctor) and documented on the LCP.

In addition, a registered doctor involved in the patients care will need to complete the Medical Certificate of Cause of Death. This will only be completed if the death was expected, as in the case of patients who die supported by the LCP, and the doctor is confident of the cause of death.

Relatives must be given formal notice that the medical certificate has been signed and informed of the procedures for its collection. On some occasions the doctor will verify and certify the death at the same time, on other occasions depending on the circumstances, a health professional will verify the death and the patient's doctor will certify the death later, for instance at a funeral director's premises if the patient died at home. This medical certificate is required to enable the family to register the death and make funeral arrangements. In the UK a death has to be registered within five days at the Registry of Births, Deaths, and Marriages office in the area where the deceased has died.

Doctors who certify an expected death should have treated the patient during their illness and visited them at least two weeks prior to their death. Should this not be the case, a doctor will need to report the death to the Coroner. This can be particularly distressing for the family and it should be explained that this is a 'formality', which may or may not result in a post-mortem. A death may be reported to the Coroner for other reasons, for instance occupational diseases, or if the doctor has concerns about the cause of death. If the Coroner decides a post-mortem is necessary, the family need to be informed and given the reason why. It is advisable to inform the family to contact the Coroner's office direct for further information. If the deceased is to be cremated, then in addition to the medical certificate of cause of death, a separate cremation form has to be completed by two independent doctors.

Saying goodbye and viewing the deceased

Many bereaved relatives welcome and value the opportunity to view their loved ones. Seeing the body is an important part of the adjustment process as it provides an opportunity to see and become familiar with the realities of death, to say a last goodbye and perhaps hold someone close for the last time. However, others may have clear feelings that they do not wish to view the body and wish to remain with memories of their loved one. For those who do wish to view the body, the thought of, or the actual experience of seeing a dead body may be very frightening, particularly if they have had no previous experience. Thus, viewing the deceased may present nurses with practical problems as the relatives may become more openly emotional and acutely distressed. This in turn may require an increased emotional input in addition to continuing with ongoing work demands (32).

When viewing the body, the bereaved should be supported by someone previously known to the patient and family. It is important to allocate some dedicated time with the bereaved. Ideally the venue should be private, quiet, and free of interruptions. Where this is not possible, the family should be asked if they are comfortable conversing in this setting (3,36–38). Acknowledgement of 'less than perfect surroundings' often reassures family members of the professional's understanding of the situation and any steps taken to communicate information well, will minimize the impact on the family and facilitate positive coping.

It can be difficult communicating with the bereaved immediately after a death as there are no 'right' words to say. Showing genuine concern, empathy, active listening, and acknowledging their concerns can help the bereaved to express their feelings of loss. It can be helpful to acknowledge their pain and say words such as 'I'm sorry for your loss', 'is there anything you need', 'is there anything I can do for you right now'.

It is helpful to explain how the deceased may look after death. Changes to their appearance should be sensitively highlighted in advance, such as colour and temperature, as the relatives maybe affected by the deceased's appearance. Use of words to describe how the body might feel and look, such as 'cold', 'may appear to be asleep' can be helpful.

The bereaved should be escorted when viewing. Some relatives prefer time alone with the deceased, others may wish to be with someone as it can be comforting not to be alone. It is important that throughout this viewing, relatives know that they can touch and speak to the deceased if they so wish. Depending where the viewing is taking place, it may be possible, if the family wishes to have a member of the clergy, priest, or faith advisor to visit and pray with them.

When the relatives have said their goodbyes it is courteous to check whether there is anything more that they need help with. Guidance should be given on what to do next and what they need to be thinking about over the next few days.

Communicating with the bereaved relatives allows professionals to consider whether any individuals are considered to be particularly vulnerable. It is essential to document clearly the main content of any discussions and the family's responses in the documentation. Any key concerns should be forwarded to the deceased family's doctor with the relative's consent. This allows the doctor the opportunity to provide further support to the family, and provides continuity of bereavement care with signposting and referral to further support as appropriate.

Information needs

Goal 11 of the LCP focuses on providing information for relatives in order that they have an understanding of what to do next. Immediately after a death, it is difficult for the bereaved to absorb the necessary information. Verbal information should be supported with appropriate clear, simple written information.

This information may include what to do after a death, advice and support on coping with bereavement, and where to turn for help including contact details for bereavement services and other help agencies. Although the majority of people will not need ongoing help, written information about grief and support services should always be provided (10).

In conclusion caring for the deceased and bereaved adults immediately before and after death is often one of the most difficult and challenging aspects of professional practice.

When this aspect of care is done well it can help families manage their situation positively, reduce the potential additional burden or upset that poor care and communication can cause, and prevent complicated grief reactions occurring.

Further resources

http://healthguides.mapofmedicine.com/choices/map/death_and_bereavement1.html
   Map of Medicine Healthguides provides an evidence-based pathway for death and bereavement.

http://www.crusebereavementcare.org.uk Cruse Bereavement Care provides counselling and support, and offers information, advice, education, and training services.

http://www.bereavementadvice.org Offers advice on all aspects of bereavement, from registering the death and finding a funeral director through to probate, tax, and benefit queries.

http://www.facingbereavement.co.uk Provides online information such as arranging a funeral, memorials, emotional issues, and financial matters.

http://www.direct.gov.uk/en/Governmentcitizensandrights/index.htm A government website providing information about practical and emotional aspects of death and bereavement.

References

1 Hills M, Albarran JW. Evaluating last offices care to improve services for newly bereaved relatives. *Nurs Times*, 2009;**105**(23):14–16

2 World Health Organization. *WHO definition of palliative care*. Available at: http://www.who.int/cancer/palliative/definition/en/ (accessed 17 November 2009)

3 National Institute for Clinical Excellence NICE (2004). *Improving supportive and palliative care for adults with cancer*. NICE, London

4 Department of Health (2008). *End of Life Care Strategy–Promoting high quality care for all adults at the end of life*. Department of Health, London

5 Scottish Government (2008). *Living and Dying Well: A national action plan for palliative and end of life care in Scotland*. Scottish Government, Edinburgh

6 Parkes CM (1993). Bereavement as a psychosocial transition: Process of adaption to change, in Stroebe MS, Stroebe W, Hansson RO (eds) *Handbook of bereavement, theory, research and intervention*, 91–101. Cambridge University Press, New York

7 Bonanno GA, Kaltman S. The varieties of grief experience. *Clin Psychol Rev* 2001;**21**(5):705–34

8 Jacobs S, Ostfeld A. An epidemiological review of the mortality of bereavement. *Psychosom Med*, 1997;**39**(5):344–57.

9 Stroebe MS, Hansson RO, Stroebe W, Schut H (2001). Introduction: Concepts and issues in contemporary research on bereavement, in Stroebe MS, Hansson RO, Stroebe W, Schut H (eds) *Handbook of bereavement research: Consequences, coping, and care*, 3–22. American Psychological Association, Washington

10 Relf M, Machin L, Archer N (2008). *Guidance for bereavement needs assessment in palliative care*. Help the Hospices, London

11 Stroebe W, Schut H (2001). Risk factors in bereavement outcome: A methodological and empirical review, in Stroebe MS, Hansson RO, Stroebe W, Schut H (eds) *Handbook of bereavement research: Consequences, coping, and care*, 349–71. American Psychological Association, Washington

12 Field D, Copp G. Communication and awareness about dying in the 1990s. *Palliat Med*, 1999;**13**(6):459–68.

13 Relf M (2008). Risk assessment and adult bereavement services, in Payne S, Seymore J, Ingleton C (eds) *Palliative care nursing. Principles and evidence for practice*, 2nd ed. 473–88. McGraw Open University Press, Berkshire

14 Aranda S, Milne D (2000). *Guidelines for the assessment of complicated bereavement risk in family members of people receiving palliative care*. Centre for Palliative Care, Melbourne

15 Kissane D (2008). Bereavement support services, in Payne S, Seymore J, Ingleton C (eds) *Palliative care nursing. Principles and evidence for practice*, 2nd ed. 489–506. McGraw Open University Press, Berkshire

16 Payne SA, Relf M. The assessment of need for bereavement follow-up in palliative and hospice care. *Palliat Med*, 1994;**8**:291–7

17 Field D, Reid D, Payne SA, Relf M. . Survey of UK hospice and specialist palliative care adult bereavement services. *Int J Palliat Nurs*, 2004;**10**(12):569–76

18 Stroebe M, Folkman S, Hansson R, Schut H. The prediction of bereavement outcome: development of an integrative risk factor framework. *Soc Sci Med*, 2006;**63**:2440–51.

19 Costello J. The emotional cost of palliative care. *Eur J Palliat Care*, 1996;**3**(4):171–74.

20 Clukey L. Anticipatory mourning: processes of expected loss in palliative care. *Int J Palliat Nurs*, 2008;**14**(7):316–25.

21 Lindemann E. The symptomatology and management of acute grief. *Am JPsychiatry*, 1944;**101**:141–48.

22 Schoenberg B, Carr AC, Kutscher AH, Peretz D, Goldberg IK (Eds) (1974). *Anticipatory grief*. Columbia University Press, New York

23 Rando TA (Ed) (1986). *Anticipatory grief and loss*. Research press, Lexington Massachusetts

24 Glick IO, Weiss RS, Parkes CM (1974). *The first year of bereavement*. J. Wiley and sons, New York

25 Evans AJ. Anticipatory grief: a theoretical challenge. *Palliat Med* 1994;**8**:159–65

26 Machin L (2001). *Exploring a framework for understanding the range of response to loss; a study of clients receiving bereavement counselling.* Keele University [Unpublished PhD thesis], *cited in* Relf M, Machin L, Archer N (2008) *Guidance for bereavement needs assessment in palliative care.* Help the Hospices, London

27 Parkes C, Laugani P, Young B (1997). *Death and bereavement across cultures.* Routledge, London

28 Payne S (2008). Loss and bereavement: Overview, in Payne S, Seymore J, Ingleton C (eds) *Palliative care nursing. Principles and evidence for practice*, 2nd ed. 425–48. McGraw Open University Press, Berkshire

29 Costello J (2004). *Nursing the dying patient. Caring in different contexts.* Palgrave Macmillan, Hampshire

30 Kent H, McDowell J. Sudden bereavement in acute care settings. *Nurs Stand*, 2004;**19**(6):38–42

31 Quested B, Rudge T. Nursing care of dead bodies: a discursive analysis of last offices. *Journal of Advanced Nursing*, 2003;**41**(6):553–60

32 Haas F. Bereavement care: Seeing the body. *Nurs Stand*, 2003;**17**(28):33–37

33 Cleiren MPHD, Van Zoelen AJ. Post-mortem organ donation and grief: A study of consent, refusal and well-being in bereavement. *Death Studies*, 2002;**26**(10):837–49.

34 National Health Service. *NHS Blood and Transplant NHSBT.* Available at: http://www.nhsbt.nhs.uk/ (accessed 22 December 2009)

35 National Health Service. *NHS Blood and Transplant NHSBT.* Available at: http://www.uktransplant.org.uk/ (accessed 22 December 2009)

36 Waller S, Dewar S, Masterson A, Finn H (2008). Improving environments for end of life care: lessons learnt from eight UK pilot sites. King's Fund, London

37 Department of Health (2006). *Care and respect in death: Good practice guidance for NHS mortuary staff.* Department of Health, London

38 Department of Health (2005). *When a patient dies: Advice on developing bereavement services in the NHS.* Department of Health, London (accessed 6 February 2010)

Chapter 8

Supporting children as death approaches and afterwards

Barbara Monroe

The death of someone significant is a challenging experience for any child or young person. However, many countries, including the UK, do not collect national statistics about prevalence. A recent secondary analysis of the 2004 'Mental health of children and young people in Great Britain' data (1), indicates that about 3.5% of those currently aged 5–16 have been bereaved of a parent or sibling, with 6.3% experiencing the death of a close friend (2). A study by Harrison and Harrington suggested that 78% of young people report bereavement of a close or significant relationship before the age of 16 (3). Holland reported that 70% of primary schools in the UK will be dealing with a recently bereaved child at any one time (4). These estimates suggest that bereavement is a much more common experience for children than we may wish to believe. What is clear is that adults' fear and silence can leave children's grief invisible and unsupported. Loss and death are part of life and however strong our desire to protect children, we cannot create for them a world in which these experiences do not exist. Children are always aware when something significant is happening in the family and if communication is missing or inadequate, they may be left alone with their fears and fantasies. Children overhear conversations, are aware of practical changes, observe body language and often pick up adult gossip from young friends. They will have concerns about whether they are to blame in some way and will wonder what is going to happen to them and to others they care about if no one speaks to them. Without dialogue they cannot be offered support with their sadness or their anxieties. Helping children to confront and learn about death and grief can assist them to develop emotional capacities that will support them for their rest of their lives. Health and social care professionals have an important role in supporting parents and families to help their children.

The impact of bereavement upon children

Some children will be bereaved through sudden death such as road traffic collision, heart attack, or stroke. Others will be bereaved through terminal illness, thus providing an opportunity to offer support before the death and for children to gain some understanding of and be involved in the dying process. Research in the area is sparse but Pfeffer's work suggests that children who have had some preparation for a death, experience less psychological difficulties than those whose parents die suddenly (5). Siegel and colleagues examined the psychological adjustment of children with a terminally ill parent and noted that these children had higher levels of self reported depression and anxiety and lower self esteem than those of a community sample (6). They subsequently reported that children's levels of depression and anxiety were higher before the death than after the death (7). This suggestion that the terminal phase of parent's illness may be a time of greater vulnerability for children than after the death, is underlined by Christ's study of 88 families where a parent was dying (8). 157 children were involved in the study and reported high stress during the terminal illness with a decrease in levels after the death. Most children returned to the same level of functioning as they had pre death (83%) and those who did not, often had a series of additional stressors after the death such as moving house, mental ill health in a surviving parent, or poverty. Christ's study refers to the 'cascade of events' that children can experience consequent upon a death. Family dynamics will change and children may find themselves taking on new routines and responsibilities or having to move house or school. Many children also report anxieties about changing relationships with their friends who may feel embarrassed and uncertain about how to respond to their bereavement. Christ's work also indicated that efforts to support parents during the illness yielded benefits for their children. Helping parents to understand their children's needs and developmental stage improved parenting competence.

The importance of the psychological wellbeing of the surviving parent or carer and their ability to continue to parent their child in bereavement, has emerged as a very significant influence on the outcome of children's bereavement (9,10). The Harvard Child Bereavement Study used a non clinical sample of 125 bereaved children with a matched control group of non bereaved children and followed them for 2 years following the death of a parent (11). Importantly both children and adults were used as respondents. The study emphasized that for a child the death of someone significant is not a single stressful event but a series of events occurring both before and after the death. Multiple variables played out over time were likely to increase or lessen the individual's vulnerability to developing social or emotional difficulties. Apart from the overriding importance of parenting capacity, other mediators included: the relationship of the child with the deceased parent, the extent of support from peers and others outside the family, characteristics of the child themselves and their prior experiences of loss, and broader structural issues such as material circumstances, class, and gender. About one third of the children experienced serious emotional or behavioural difficulties at some point during the two years of the study. The percentage of bereaved children in the high risk group exceeded that for controls. A recent study by Cerel of over 360 parentally bereaved children found a link with increased psychiatric symptomology in children and that those children whose surviving parent had high levels of depression in the presence of other stressful life events were at higher risk (12). All these studies suggest that giving parents information about their children's needs at the time of a death and supporting them to involve their children can benefit children's subsequent adjustment.

Ribbens McCarthy's thorough review indicates that the evidence for a direct association between bereavement and negative outcomes in terms of social adjustment and mental health is both complex and contradictory (13). For example some bereaved children appear to achieve more highly educationally, where others appear to lose motivation and confidence. Some report an increase in self esteem, others higher levels of depression and anxiety. Most studies have methodical weaknesses. However, when bereavement is experienced alongside other difficulties and pre existing vulnerabilities, the evidence is stronger for greater risk of poor outcomes (14). Increased risks appear to centre around issues of health, self esteem, educational achievement, and the risk of increased disruptive behaviour such as aggression, involvement in criminal offences, drug taking, and early sexual experiences. There is some evidence of a link to poor care and sometimes abuse (15). A crucial issue for individual responses to a death is the meaning the relationship had in the child's life. The death of a distant grandparent will have a very different impact to the death of a grandparent who was a daily carer of a child. Another important consideration is the very long periods of time over which bereavement may continue to affect children and young people, as their understanding and appreciation of their loss changes as they themselves develop. They re-visit their grief, expressing and experiencing it in different ways, especially at times of future transition or loss (16,17).

How do we help parents to help their children?

There are good reasons for parental reluctance to involve children when someone significant in the family is dying. Many parents are anxious about managing their own feelings and have unvoiced concerns about being overwhelmed by the child's grief. Adults may be concerned about what their child may or may not know already and about how to use vocabulary and explanations they will understand. Other members of the extended family may be suggesting that children are too young to be told or that now is not the right time. Everyone will be worrying about making things worse. Macpherson's study of the impact of terminal illness on the well parent emphasizes the difficulty of dealing with uncertainty (18). Participants spoke of knowing that the death would happen but needing to deny it and of the exhaustion of controlling overwhelming feelings of sadness, fear, and anger, whilst trying to avoid their partner feeling a burden. Partners who cannot share information between themselves and discuss their feelings together may find it difficult to talk to their children. The first task may be to help them to talk to one another.

In the few studies where children and young people have been asked directly about what they want, most have seemed clear that they would like to have information. Beale found that children with dying parents experienced distress but also had a greater understanding of the illness than is usually suspected (19). The study suggested that children's increased anxiety is often linked to a lack of information or a chance to talk it through. Chowns' small participative enquiry with young people who had a parent with terminal illness indicated clearly that they were not just passive recipients of adult interventions (20). All nine young people wanted to be told the truth as soon as possible and to be involved. They actively sought out information and were clearly selecting what they saw as appropriate coping strategies for different eventualities. They tried to support their parents and wanted respect for their own competence. At the same time it was clear that coping with uncertainty was frustrating and frightening. Studies also indicate that children value the opportunity to ask doctors questions about what is happening or has happened (21,22). These studies also reinforce clinical experience that children want to protect their parents and often attempt to obey family rules even if they are unwritten. If the family emotional atmosphere is saying, 'We don't talk about it, don't ask'; children may try to join in the pretence that nothing is happening. Professionals must not join the conspiracy of silence and should make a direct offer of help, 'A lot of parents worry about their children at times like this and I wonder if it would help to talk'. However, professionals must not take over from parents. Parents are the experts on their children and will be around long after the professionals have disappeared. Professionals should work in a family context, respecting parents and carers and offering them encouragement; working with what they can manage rather than implying there is a recipe which if followed will improve children's chances (23). For example, if a parent cannot face their child going to the funeral, they could be encouraged to think about an alternative such as the children going to a close friend's house and to think about how to mark the occasion for them, perhaps visiting the crematorium or cemetery

> ## Box 8.1 What do children need?
>
> ◆ Respect and acknowledgement
> ◆ Clear, simple, truthful information about what is happening and why
>   and what might happen next
> ◆ Reassurance about practical issues and about their own future care
> ◆ Reassurance that nothing they did or said made the illness happen
> ◆ The opportunity to talk about feelings with adults who are prepared to
>   share their own
> ◆ A chance to be involved in helping the patient
>   and subsequently:
> ◆ The chance to tell the story of what has happened
> ◆ Support to cope with changed circumstances
> ◆ Help to remember together

together at a later time, taking photographs of floral tributes, or showing a child letters of condolence. Box 8.1 lists what children need near the time of their parent's death.

Helping parents to talk to their children

It is important to recognize parents' own feelings and to acknowledge that this is one of the most difficult things that any parent has to do and that it will feel very uncomfortable. We can remind parents that any conversation is just an opening. Bite sized chunks of information are important; not everything has to be said at one time. Parents should be warned not to be surprised if children then change the subject or focus on something practical like what they are going to have for tea. It generally helps to start by finding out what the child knows or believes about what is happening and to link explanations to things that children have noticed already. *'What have you noticed that is different about mummy?'* This gives the opportunity to correct any misapprehensions and to validate the child's experience. At a minimum, children will need to know that the person is very ill indeed and what the illness is called. Parents may be helped by being forewarned about typical questions from children: *'Can I catch the illness? Did I cause it? Will the person die? Will anyone else die? Who will look after me? Who will do the things that the dying person did?'* All parents need reassurance that it is alright to say: *'I don't know; That's a difficult question; I don't know the answer right now; We will need to get some more information; Perhaps the doctor can help us.*' Parents should try to avoid making promises that cannot be kept. It is not helpful to say, *'No one else in the family will die,'* but it is possible to say, *'It's very unusual for someone as young as mummy to be so ill that the doctors can't help to get her better'*.

Giving information

Parents may value suggestions of words to use and possible explanations and may then want to talk to their children alone. Others may welcome the support of doctors and nurses in explaining details about an illness to their children. Having appropriate leaflets available for parents about their children's needs so that they can think about issues in advance is very helpful. Children should not be pushed to talk or frightened with excessive medical detail. Young children have short time concepts and explanations should proceed gradually: *'Daddy is now so ill the doctors cannot make him better, but together we can do all sorts of things to keep him comfortable'*; *'Daddy is now so ill we don't think he will live much longer'*; *'Daddy is now very weak and we know that he will die'*. Parents will inevitably be distressed and children can be helped by being told when something is painful. *'It is hard for me talk about this because it makes me feel sad, but we will always love one another.'* Explanations about what is happening as it happens are reassuring, and sharing feelings helps children learn about grief and gives them permission to talk to their parents about their own feelings.

Being present and being involved

If the dying person is unconscious children can still be present at the bedside for short periods. *'Even if mummy can't talk to you we think she can still probably hear and will know that you are here. She will always love you. You can hold her hand.'* If children do not wish to visit they can be encouraged to send a card or drawing. Even a very short visit can help the child to feel involved and will be remembered later. It is always important to enquire about belief systems and to respect family culture. However, simple factual explanations of death are helpful to children and euphemisms should be avoided, for example linking death with sleep and journeys can be confusing. *'When somebody is dead, their body has stopped working. It is not like being asleep. When somebody is dead, their body cannot wake up, it has stopped working forever. It will never eat, drink, feel sad or happy again and it cannot feel pain.'*

When death is unexpected

It will be important, although difficult, to ask whoever is present whether there are any children likely to be closely affected by this death. If it is a very close relationship such as a parent, those relatives present may need support and help to arrange for a child to visit whatever the time of day or night. Equally, the only thing possible may be to talk through with a parent or carer what they will say to the child on their return home. Sudden death makes it much harder for children to believe what has happened especially if there has been no chance to say goodbye. Parents will need suggestions of possible explanations, '*I have something very sad to tell you. Your sister was coming home and crossing the road when a lorry came round the corner and knocked her over. She hurt her head very badly. When she got to the hospital they said that she was already dead. She had been too badly hurt to be made better.*' Children can cope with difficult information if they know they are cared for and they will feel valued when an attempt is made to talk to them even if the words come out wrong.

There may sometimes be immediate concerns about who will have parental responsibility for a child subsequent to the death, particularly where there are complex re-constituted family circumstances. It will then be important to encourage families to get advice from a solicitor and if possible to involve a social worker. Parents may also need particular support where a child has a disability such as a learning disability (24).

Viewing the body

Viewing the body can help a child to begin to accept what has happened. If they are forbidden to do so they may imagine something much more frightening than the reality or think that they are not important enough to be included. They will however need preparation if they are to make a proper choice. They will need to know what the room will look like, that the body will be cold and that they will be accompanied by someone they know and trust. '*We can see grand-dad's body at the funeral directors. They will have put him in a special box called a coffin but we will be able to see his face. His eyes will be closed. He will feel cold because they have to keep his body in a fridge until the funeral.*' If children decide to view they may need explicit permission to touch the body or put something personal in the coffin.

Attending funerals

After a death, some parents may be anxious about whether or not their children should attend the funeral. It is important to remind parents that funerals are family occasions. Not being able to take part in saying goodbye to the person who has died can make it harder to accept the death and to start grieving. Most children will not have been to a funeral before and will need some explanations. '*A funeral is a special time when all the people who knew grand-dad will come together to remember him and to say goodbye. There will be prayers and music and special readings.'* Many parents worry about how old children should be before they go to a funeral. Children who are old enough to go to school have learnt to sit still and concentrate for short periods. Younger children will need to be reassured that someone will be there who will go outside with them if they find it too difficult. Parents are often helped by a reminder that this person does not have to be them. They can ask someone who knows the child well and who is not as closely involved as they are. Children can be helped to feel part of the funeral by choosing a reading, a hymn or special flowers. If they have chosen not to go or if parents do not want them to be there, it is important to remind parents that they need to tell the children as soon as possible about what happened at the funeral so they do not feel left out.

Children's understanding of death

Research indicates that children acquire death concepts in stages, moving from the concrete, e.g. 'dead bodies don't move', to the abstract, 'everybody will die one day' (25). Younger children, particularly those under the age of five sometimes see death as reversible and often have 'magical thinking'. They may feel that they have caused the death through something they did or said. They need explicit reassurance that this is not so. They can upset parents with constant questions such as, '*Is daddy coming home tomorrow?*' and will need simple information repeated over and over again. It helps to warn parents of this possibility. A study by Lansdowne and Benjamin suggests that many children of five or six years old have a clear understanding of death (26) and Silverman emphasizes that even very young children can be helped to understand by being given clear explanations in age appropriate language (27). Way underlines the importance of very young children, who are perhaps babies when somebody dies, being given information as they develop language so that they can create memories and integrate the story of the dead person into their own ongoing lives (28).

Subsequent support

There has been much debate about whether or not all bereaved children need support and when and what kind of support should be offered if deemed necessary. Harrington and Harrison emphasize the lack of evidence about the benefits of the very varied services available (29). There are significant difficulties in evaluating the efficacy of preventive interventions (30) and there has been criticism of outcome measures based solely on psychiatric morbidity (31). However, Sandler and colleagues' meticulous evaluation of a family bereavement programme aimed at improving family functioning demonstrated positive outcomes (32). Nabors studied children who had attended a 'grief camp' and the respondents said that it had been helpful to be with other children in similar circumstances and to be able to express their feelings (33). The Childhood Bereavement Network, the UK federation of childhood bereavement services declares that 'all children and young people, together with their families and other care givers'. . . should be able to . . . 'easily access a choice of high quality local and national information, guidance, and support to enable them to manage the impact of death on their lives'(34). It is hard to disagree with this. Only a few children will need intensive therapy and effective referral routes should be present to secure support for those who require it. All parents should be given simple written information about ongoing sources of support and many will value advice about what behaviours to expect and when to worry. Things to be concerned about are: ongoing nightmares and sleep problems that affect daily life, for example meaning that children cannot go to school; children persistently refusing to go to school and withdrawing from usual activities and interests; or exhibiting unusually aggressive behaviour on an ongoing basis. Equally many children may become more clingy, more naughty, or unusually quiet and well behaved, or exhibit increased somatic symptoms as part of normal reactions to loss. The key is the severity and longevity of responses rather than their presence alone.

Children need support to remember

Parents will need reassurance that it is alright to cry in front of children who learn how to grieve by watching adults do it. Children can also be helped to understand that grief brings difficult feelings, '*I am sorry I was cross today. I am not angry with you, I am just missing Mummy a lot*'. It will also help if rules and routines stay as consistent as possible. It helps if children have something that belonged to the person who died. They will need opportunities to remember together with others in their family. '*Do you remember when we were all on holiday together? Let's look at the photographs.*' Children may want to put a special photograph in a frame, to light a candle on special occasions or to make a memory box. There are now several interactive websites for older children to share feelings and anxieties. Parents may need to be reminded that they do not have to do everything themselves and that others can help. School is an important source of normality and support for many children and parents may value discussing how to approach teachers. Above all parents need reassuring that children are resilient and, with support, will cope with the challenges of loss.

Further resources

Winston's Wish (2007). *As Big as it Gets—supporting a child when a parent is seriously ill.* Winston's Wish, Cheltenham. A booklet for parents.

www.winstonswish.org.uk Includes an interactive website for young people; and also runs a national telephone helpline.

Candle (2005). *Children and funerals.* St Christopher's Hospice, London. A booklet for parents.

Social Work Dept, St Christopher's Hospice (1989). *Someone special has died.* St Christopher's Hospice, London (a booklet for children).

www.riprap.org.uk. For young people with a parent who has cancer.

www.crusebereavementcare.org.uk. Can offer referrals to Cruse branches throughout the country.

www.uk-sobs.org.uk. For survivors of bereavement by suicide.

www.childhoodbereavementnetwork.org.uk. A national federation of children's bereavement services with a directory of locally available services for bereaved children and their families

www.childbereavement.org.uk. Resources and information for children and families and training for professionals.

MCPCIL. Supporting children and their families within the Liverpool Care Pathway for the Dying Patient (LCP) Programme www.mcpcil.org.uk/liverpool-care-pathway/ documentation-lcp.htm#supporting%20children (last accessed 30th August 2010).

References

1 Green H et al. (2005) *Mental Health of Children and Young People in Great Britain 2004.* HMSO, London.

2 Fauth B, Thompson M, Penny A. (2009) *Associations between childhood bereavement and children's background, experiences and outcomes.* National Children's Bureau, London.

3 Harrison L, Harrington R. Adolescents' bereavement experiences. Prevalence, association with depressive symptoms and use of services. *J Adolesc* 2001;**24** (2):159–69.

4 Holland J. Child bereavement in Humberside primary schools. *Educational Research*, 1993;**35**(3):289–97.

5 Pfeffer C, Karus D, Siegel K. Child survivors of parental death from cancer or suicide: depressive behavioural outcomes. *Psycho-oncology* 2000;**9**:1–10.

6 Siegel K, Mesagno FP, Karus D, Christ G, Banks K, Moynihan R. Psychosocial adjustment of children with a terminally ill parent. *J Am Acad Child Adolesc Psychiatry* 1992:**31**(2):327–33.

7 Seigel K, Raveis VH, Karus D (1996). Pattern of communication with children when a parent has cancer. In: Baider L, Cooper CL, De-Nour AK (eds), *Cancer and the family.* 109–29. John Wiley and Sons, Chichester.

8 Christ G (2000). *Healing children's grief; surviving a parent's death from cancer.* Oxford University Press, New York.

9 Harris T, Brown GW, Bifulco A. Loss of parent in childhood and adult psychiatric disorder: the role of lack of adequate parental care. *Psychol Med* 1986;**16**:641–59.

10 Christ GH, Christ AE. Current approaches to helping children cope with a parent's terminal illness. *CA Cancer J Clin* 2006;**56**:197–212.

11 Worden JW (1996). *Children and grief: when a parent dies*. Guilford Press, New York.

12 Cerel J, Fristad M, Verducci J, Weller RA, Weller EB. Childhood bereavement: Psychopathology in the 2 years post parental death. *J Am Acad Child Adolesc Psychiatry* 2006;**45**(6):681–90.

13 Ribbens McCarthy J (2006) *Young people's experiences of loss and bereavement: towards an interdisciplinary approach*. Open University Press, Berkshire, UK.

14 Ribbens McCarthy J (2007) *Highlight no 232: Children, Young People and Bereavement*. National Children's Bureau, London.

15 Cross S (2002) *I can't stop feeling sad: calls to ChildLine about bereavement*. ChildLine Special Report. ChildLine, London.

16 Lohnes K, Kalter N. Preventative intervention groups for parentally bereaved children. *Am J Orthopsychiatry* 1994;**64**:594–603.

17 Christ G. (2006). Providing a home–based therapeutic program for widows and children. In: Green P, Kane G, Christ G, Lynch S and Corrigan M. (eds) *FDNY crisis counselling: Innovative responses to 9/11 firefighters, families and communities*. 180–211. Wiley Publishing, New York.

18 Macpherson C. Telling children their ill parent is dying: a study of the factors influencing the well parent. *Mortality* 2005;**10**(2):113–126.

19 Beale EA, Sivesind D, Bruera E. Parents dying of cancer and their children. *Palliat Support Care* 2004;**2**:387–93.

20 Chowns G. End of life care discussions–but not in front of the children? *End of Life Care* 2009;**3**(1):42–47.

21 Monroe B, Kraus F. Children and loss. *Br J Hosp Med* 1996;**56**:260–4.

22 Thompson F, Payne S. Bereaved children's questions to a doctor. *Mortality* 2000;**5**: 74–96.

23 Monroe B, Sheldon F. (2004) Psychosocial dimensions of care. In: Sykes N, Edmonds P, Wiles J. (eds) *Management of advanced disease* (4th ed.) 405–38 Arnold, London.

24 McEnhill L. (2009) Loss for children with learning disability. In: Monroe B, Kraus F (eds). *Brief Interventions with Bereaved Children* (2nd ed.) 121–28. Oxford University Press, Oxford.

25 Dyregrov A. (2008) *Grief in children: a handbook for adults*. (2nd ed.). Jessica Kingsley, London.

26 Lansdown R, Benjamin C. The development of the concept of death in children aged 5-9. *Child Care Health Dev* 1985;**11**:13–20.

27 Silverman P (2000). *Never too young to know*. Oxford University Press, New York.

28 Way P. (2009) Co-creating memory: supporting very young children. In: Monroe B, Kraus F (eds) *Brief Interventions with Bereaved Children* (second ed) 129–34. Oxford University Press, Oxford.

29 Harrington R, Harrison L. Unproven assumptions about the impact of bereavement on children. *J R Soc Med* 1999;**92**:230–3.

30 Christ G, Raveis V, Siegel K, Karus D, Christ A. Evaluation of a preventive intervention for bereaved children. *J Soc Work End Life Palliat Care*, 2005;**1**(3):57–81.

31 Stokes J, Pennington J, Monroe B, Papadatou D, Relf M. Developing services for bereaved children: a discussion of the theoretical and practical issues involved. *Mortality*, 1999;**4**(3): 291–307.

32 Sandler I et al. The family bereavement program: efficacy evaluation *J of Consulting and Clinical Psychology*, 2003;**71**(3):587–600.

33 Nabors L, Ohms M, Buchanan N, Kirsh KL, Nash T, Passik SD, Johnson JL, Snapp J Brown G. A pilot study of the impact of a grief camp for children. *Palliat Support Care* 2004;**2**:403–8

34 Penny A. (2009). Childhood bereavement: the context and need for services. In: Monroe B, Kraus F (eds). *Brief Interventions with Bereaved Children* (2nd ed.) 10. Oxford University Press, Oxford.

Chapter 9

Induction and implementation of the Liverpool Care Pathway for the Dying Patient

Maureen Gambles, Anita Roberts, and Rita Doyle

Introduction

Over the past few years a major drive has been underway to ensure that the care of all dying patients and their relatives or carers is of the highest possible standard in the last hours or days of their lives. The Liverpool Care Pathway for the Dying Patient (LCP) Continuous Quality Improvement Programme was recognized in England as a model of best practice in the NHS Beacon Programme (2001) (1) and was subsequently incorporated into the Cancer Services Collaborative Project and the National End of Life Care Programme (2). It was recommended in the NICE guidance on supportive and palliative care for patients with cancer as a mechanism for identifying and addressing the needs of dying patients (3). It was recommended in the Department of Health White Paper of 2006 (4) as a tool that should be rolled out across England and is also recommended in the Department of Health End of Life Care Strategy (5) and highlighted in the Department of Health End of Life Care Quality Markers document (6).

The LCP model aims to improve care of the dying by expanding the knowledge base related to the process of dying to improve the quality of care delivered in the last hours or days of life. The LCP generic version 12 document guides and enables healthcare professionals to focus on care in the last hours or days of life. This aims to provide high quality care tailored to the patient's individual needs, when their death is expected. It is in no way meant to replace the skill and expertise of the practitioner using it, but it does require clinicians to decide the focus of care for each individual patient at this time. Where specific goals of care are deemed not to be in the best interest of an individual patient, practitioners are encouraged to fully document their reasons for this. Using the LCP involves regular assessment of the patient's condition requiring continuous reflection, challenge, critical decision making, and clinical skill.

There are five key areas that are vital to the safe and successful implementation and sustainability of the programme within any environment: clinical decision making, management and leadership, learning and teaching, research and development, and governance and risk. It is only possible to use the LCP document successfully when the organization and health care professionals working within it have embraced these areas in their entirety as part of the drive for continuous quality improvement.

The LCP document has itself been subject to a continuous cycle of review and revision since its inception in the late 1990s. In 2009, LCP generic version 12 was published following a two year comprehensive consultation process and incorporating the latest findings and evidence base from two National Care of the Dying Audit Hospitals (NCDAH) (7).

This chapter outlines the various elements of the LCP document and the process through which successful implementation of the LCP for care in the last hours or days of life can be achieved using the 10 step Continuous Quality Improvement Programme. Aspects that are fundamental throughout the 10 step programme, such as education and training and the use of local audit to promote quality assurance will be explained.

Implementing the LCP

The key aims of the LCP induction and implementation programme are to:

+ Improve the care of patients in the last hours or days of life
+ Improve the experience of the relative or carer during this period and into bereavement
+ Empower generic workers
+ Demonstrate outcomes of care
+ Promote care of the dying as a quality indicator at governance and management level.

The Deming or Plan, Do, Study, Act (PDSA) cycle illustrates the key methodology used in implementing change and is recommended by the LCP Central Team as a model for implementation of the LCP. There are four stages to the Deming (PDSA) cycle (8):

Plan: agree the change to be implemented

Do: carry out the change and measure the impact

Study: study data before and after the change and reflect on learning

Act: plan the next change cycle or implementation

Any major change within an organization requires time and commitment, and implementation of the LCP is no different. The time this process takes should never be underestimated. In generic settings (e.g. hospital or community) it may take up to two years to successfully implement the LCP, whereas in specialist units like hospices, it is likely to be a much quicker process. Arguably, implementing the LCP in the care home setting poses the greatest challenge. Despite the fact that deaths frequently occur in some care homes, death and dying may not be central to care home policy which may result in the provision of relatively little end of life care education for staff. In addition, working with multiple GP practices presents a particular challenge (9). Such factors are likely to increase the time and commitment required for successful implementation in these environments.

Specific opportunities exist within the LCP programme (nationally and internationally) for organizations to receive support from the LCP Central Team for local implementation programmes. Organizations are encouraged to take advantage of these opportunities as appropriate throughout the implementation process:

- ◆ Registration with the LCP Central Team
- ◆ Base Review analysis (retrospective audit)
- ◆ Educational opportunities
- ◆ Post implementation analysis
- ◆ National audit/benchmarking

The service improvement model is a phased approach incorporating the 10 step Continuous Quality Improvement Programme for the LCP model.

Phase 1: Induction

Establishing the project (Step 1)

If the needs of people in the last hours or days of their lives are to be met, the workforce must be empowered to take a leading role in the process. Implementing the LCP effectively is one means of achieving this goal, but it requires careful planning and involves winning the hearts and minds of all involved. Implementation across a large health care setting is unlikely to succeed without first establishing meaningful change within identified pilot sites.

Key players must be identified, all relevant clinical staff involved, and executive endorsement gained at the outset. It is crucial that specialist palliative care services are involved from the outset.

LCP facilitator (lead implementer)

The identification of a key member of staff to provide leadership, and the development of a steering group to oversee the project are also essential elements for successful implementation. The use of LCP facilitators has been shown to play an important role in successful implementation (10). Evidence from the NCDAH (MCPCIL 2009) (7) suggests that having a facilitator in post is related to improved completion of the LCP document. The LCP Central Team recommends appointing a specific LCP facilitator to provide leadership for the project, to articulate and maintain a focus on the key aims of the programme and to support generic staff through this process. It is also important that the LCP facilitator (or lead implementer) takes responsibility for introducing and explaining the document and how it works to all involved. Table 9.1 illustrates potential models for LCP facilitator provision across the settings.

Registration with the LCP Central Team at the Marie Curie Palliative Care Institute Liverpool (MCPCIL)

Organizations are encouraged to register their project with the LCP Central Team as this brings a number of benefits. Support and advice on implementing

Table 9.1 Potential Models for LCP Facilitator Provision

Hospital	◆ 1 WTE/sessional LCP facilitator for approximately one year, linked with the hospital specialist palliative care service
	◆ Hospitals of 500+ beds may require more than one facilitator and/or a facilitator for up to two years
	◆ Ongoing sessional support to sustain change
Hospice	◆ Sessional commitment from an LCP facilitator for approximately 6 months
	◆ Ongoing sessional support to sustain change
Community	Depending on size of locality:
	◆ 1 WTE LCP facilitator for approximately 6–12 months linked with the community palliative care service
	◆ The role could be a joint post with a Gold Standards Framework (GSF) and/or Preferred Priorities of Care (PPC) facilitator in the UK—see end of life website www.endoflifecareforadults.nhs.uk
	◆ Ongoing sessional support to sustain change
Care Home	Depending on number of beds and number of GPs covering:
	◆ Sessional LCP facilitator for one year linked with community or hospice palliative care service
	◆ Ongoing sessional support to sustain change.

WTE: whole time equivalent

and sustaining the use of the LCP at various milestones throughout the implementation process are available to registered sites. For example, in addition to the provision of information, useful documentation, and ongoing support (telephone and email), registration with the LCP Central Team also gives access to the facility for the analysis and reporting of base review and post pathway audits which enable local implementing teams to feedback formally to staff regarding progress.

This phase is the most intensive and may take months to complete. It is pivotal to ensure this infrastructure is in place for the long term goals and sustainability of the LCP model to be realized.

Phase 2: Implementation

Development of the documentation (Step 2)

The function of the local steering group at this stage is to review the LCP document in order to assess its suitability for use locally. The prompts which support the goals on the LCP can be adapted to better reflect local practice, provided that they do not alter the meaning of the stated goals. However, no changes should be made to the wording of the stated goals of care as this may result in an inability to include these goals in any future benchmarking or national audit programmes. Should the need arise locally, extra goals may also be added to the document.

The LCP Central Team has developed the LCP Goal Definition/Data Dictionary document to explain the reason for including each goal on the LCP and to guide health care professionals to fill in the documentation appropriately (11).

The LCP Central Team is available to review each LCP and match it for compliance with the current core document so that all stakeholders have a full understanding of the similarities or differences highlighted.

The steering group also needs to consider what clinical guidance is required to support the use of the LCP and to determine where such guidance already exists, either nationally or locally, or where it needs to be developed. Symptom control protocols should be available for each of the five key symptoms that may develop in the last hours or days of life (pain, agitation, respiratory tract secretions, nausea and vomiting, and dyspnoea). It is crucial that these guidelines and protocols are agreed by the multidisciplinary team, medicines management, or appropriate equivalent within the organization. Other important issues that require the development of agreed guidance include resuscitation and skin integrity. The LCP Central Team also recommends the use of 'core' information leaflets (12):

◆ Relatives and carers information (provided as part of LCP generic version 12 document)

- Information for health care professionals (provided as part of LCP generic version 12 document)
- Facilities information (to be designed locally)
- Coping with dying leaflet (available to order via www.mcpcil.org.uk) or equivalent
- Grief and bereavement information (to be designed locally)

Retrospective audit of documentation; Base Review (Step 3)

Continuous Quality Improvement (CQI) takes a scientific approach to every-day work with the aim of improving outcomes for patient's and points out the importance of the analysis of objective data to promote quality management (13). The LCP model contains several points at which it is possible to collect, analyse, report, and reflect on objective data to gain a picture of the clinical environment.

The retrospective audit (Base Review) of the routine documentation of care given to a sample of patients in the last hours or days of life is the first opportunity to undertake such analysis and it is recommended for all organizations implementing the LCP. The LCP Central Team has produced helpful guidance notes to assist in the systematic coding of this information.

This exercise is most useful to highlight and reinforce the need for change as well as providing a baseline of performance against which to evaluate change after implementation. The base review involves organizations identifying a set of 20 recent consecutive notes from within the proposed pilot area for 'expect-ed deaths' within the environment. Whilst there is no agreed definition of 'expected death', auditors are required to identify a point in the patient record where the documentation indicates a change in the focus of care and the patient is diagnosed as dying. The information contained within the notes from this identified point in time is then scrutinized for evidence that appropriate care has been delivered in the last hours or days of life against the goals of care on the LCP. The audit also involves the collection of patient demographic information including primary diagnosis, gender, and age.

An important method for gaining support for the implementation of the LCP into any environment is inviting various members of the multidisci-plinary team in the pilot site to be involved in the Base Review process. In this way, health care professionals who often were responsible for the delivery of the care under scrutiny can experience first hand the importance of recording care delivery so that it is as consistent and comprehensive as it could or should be.

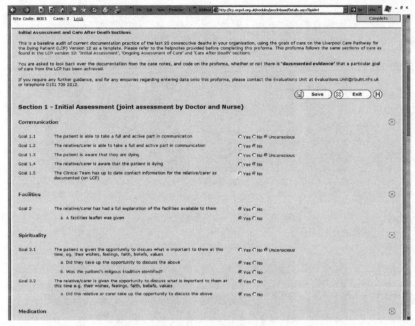

Fig. 9.1 Example of electronic data capture tool for the LCP.

An electronic data collection and reporting tool was developed to underpin the publication of the LCP generic Version 12 in November 2009. An example is shown in Figure 9.1.

The electronic tool provides a simple mechanism for entering data extracted from the notes and makes an instant report available to sites once the data has been entered and locked into the tool. The report consists mainly of simple charts and tables that illustrate where the documentation of care was achieved and where it could be improved (see Figure 9.2 for examples of the feedback routinely provided). Often the analysis illustrates that documentation of care in the last hours or days of life is poor, and so LCP facilitators are encouraged to feed back this information carefully in a way that does not demoralize staff but highlights the need for change and the opportunities for improvement provided by using the LCP.

Induction education programme (Step 4)

It is important that all staff who care for patients in the last hours or days of their lives have received appropriate education in care of the dying to underpin the safe and effective use of the LCP. The primary focus of education and training at this stage is to ensure that staff working in the pilot area(s) are able to

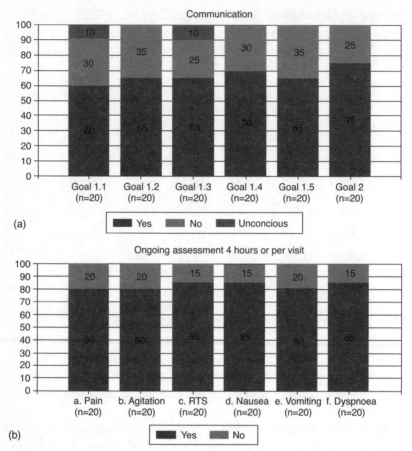

Fig. 9.2a and b Examples of electronic reports.

understand the document fully and to complete it accurately. Taking the opportunity to work through the document with small groups of staff and using the LCP Goal Definitions/Data Dictionary document to support understanding can be helpful first steps in enabling staff to become proficient in the use of the LCP.

In addition, facilitators should also work closely with their specialist palliative care colleagues to devise and deliver a locally relevant education and training programme relating to the wider issues involved in using the LCP. These are likely to include, but not necessarily be limited to, areas such as communication skills, pain and symptom control, cultural, and spiritual issues. In order to achieve this, it is important for LCP facilitators to have a good understanding of the pilot site and of the staff working within the environment. The provision of a resource folder containing relevant evidence-based documentation and guidance is recommended to support the implementation process.

The End of Life Care Strategy (5) reinforces the need for all health care professionals to have appropriate training in end of life care, including care in the last hours or days of life. It also highlights the need for clinical staff of all grades and disciplines to receive education and training in communication skills specifically for this phase of care. The Marie Curie Palliative Care Institute Liverpool is looking to further develop and evaluate a number of educational resources such as learning materials, study days, workshops, and short courses to support healthcare workers in their use of the LCP and the delivery of high quality care in the last hours or days of life. These initiatives will not only provide an excellent grounding for implementation of the LCP, but will also support this wider education and training agenda.

Clinical implementation of the LCP (Step 5)

This step begins once the relevant group of staff has received sufficient education and training (outlined above). This is likely to be the most 'hands on' phase of the project, where LCP facilitators/project leads will need to ensure that they are available within the pilot sites to offer ongoing support each time the document is used.

Maintaining a 'high profile' during this period is imperative for success, as is ensuring strong links between staff on the pilot areas and the specialist palliative care team. Liaison between staff and the LCP facilitator/specialist team each time an LCP is used is a good way to increase specific knowledge and confidence and empower health care professionals in caring for dying patients and their families.

Phase 3: Dissemination

Maintaining and improving competencies (Step 6)

Competencies should be maintained and improved by incorporating a process of ongoing review each time an LCP is used. This provides the opportunity for staff to actively engage in reflective practice. Schon suggested that the capacity to reflect on action in order to engage in a process of continuous learning was one of the defining characteristics of professional practice (14). This practice should continue at least for the first few months after the introduction of the document. Taking the opportunity to reflect formally on and discuss the specific elements of the care delivered allows the transfer and cementing of knowledge and helps to build confidence in the use of the document. Such ongoing reflection not only has the potential to highlight any inherent barriers to the delivery of optimum care, but also provides an opportunity to acknowledge and celebrate success whenever appropriate.

Learning and teaching opportunities

One of the most important factors that influences the standard of care patients receive is the quality of the skill, knowledge, and attitude of the clinicians caring for them. Organizations have a responsibility to ensure that they have the right workforce with the right skills and knowledge to deliver world class end of life care.

The majority of people (around 58%) (15) die in hospitals but evidence suggests that the majority wish to die at home. In order to redress this balance it is essential that the workforce across all care settings has the knowledge and skills to care for people effectively in the last hours or days of life. Training and education in end of life care with a particular emphasis around the LCP should be provided for all relevant staff, on a continuing basis. This is fundamental to ensuring quality in end of life care and must be a key feature across all organizations.

The LCP Central Team provides an educational programme in the form of National LCP workshops and an annual conference. This programme aims to support key staff in implementing and sustaining the use of the LCP within the clinical environment.

The National LCP workshops provide an overview of the LCP programme and the development of the LCP. Participants are given the opportunity to become familiar with the layout of LCP generic version 12 and how it should be completed. Examples from clinical practice are used to illustrate specific aspects of care. Participants are also given up to date information regarding the national end of life care agenda and wider issues including metrics, measurement, governance, and risk. The workshop examines aspects of quality, innovation, productivity, and prevention in relation to the LCP model. Participants are encouraged to identify issues relating to implementing and sustaining the LCP programme in their own clinical area.

Organizations need to develop ongoing, sustainable education and dissemination strategies. One such approach is the development of a link nurse programme. This allows lead facilitators/key champions from each clinical area using the LCP model to network and share challenges and successes.

Palliative Care Network Nurse Programme

One example of how this can be achieved is the Palliative Care Network Nurse Programme which has been running for some years within the Royal Liverpool and Broadgreen University Hospitals NHS Trust (16,17) It developed at the request of nurses who had been involved in the piloting of the LCP and has been in operation since 1999. The aim of this programme is to enhance the knowledge and skills of interested generic nurses in the palliative care approach. This is achieved through regular support from the Hospital Specialist Palliative Care Team (HSPCT) which enhances the knowledge and skills of the link nurses and enables them to take a lead role in the management of patients with end of life care needs within their clinical area, including those in the last hours or days of life. The network nurse supported by the specialist palliative care team drives the education of the clinical team in their area to promote quality care at the bedside.

The End of Life Care Strategy recognized that the delivery of high quality end of life care to individuals and their families and carers requires nothing less than a cultural shift in attitude and behaviour within the health and social care workforce(5). The network nurse plays a pivotal role in defining, and sustaining best practice across their workforce. This innovative programme directly benefits patients and their relatives or carers and translates into immense personal and professional job satisfaction for the individual nurse. The key areas of learning relate to:

- Communication skills
- Assessment and care planning
- Advance care planning
- Symptom management, comfort, and well being
- Use of the LCP

The programme specifically addresses issues such as the management of pain and other symptoms, communication and psychological support, care of the dying, and dealing with complex placement issues. Network nurses are encouraged to share their knowledge and skills (including how and when to use an LCP to support care in the last hours or days of life) with others in their immediate environment using a cascade model of teaching. Box 9.1 lists the expectations of the role of a network nurse.

In addition, four funded study days relating to the key learning areas are provided each year; each network nurse is expected to attend at least two of these per year. Each network nurse is invited to work with a named mentor from the specialist palliative care team, and participate in a Network Nurse Shadowing Programme across the community and hospice sector, where each nurse undertakes a two-day placement to enable learning about the strengths and challenges of organization and culture across care settings. The programme was subjected to a questionnaire evaluation where respondents reported that it had been beneficial, particularly in providing them with increased palliative care knowledge, and support and provided important networking opportunities (16,17).

Box 9.1 As a Palliative Care Network Nurse at the Royal Liverpool and Broadgreen University Hospital NHS Trust you will

- Be expected to take a lead role in the support and management of patients with palliative care and end of life issues on your ward. The Hospital Specialist Palliative Care Team (HSPCT) will support you to develop competencies and empower you to be able to share knowledge and skills pertaining to end of life care with other generic workers in your ward environment.

- Be expected to take responsibility for and recognize the importance of your own continuing professional development.

- Be aware of any patients who have been referred to the HSPCT and ensure that all referrals are appropriate. You should also ensure that staff are aware that the Medical Team should document their agreement for referral to the HSPCT in the patient's medical notes.

- Ensure that you monitor the care of any patient who is being cared for supported by the Liverpool Care Pathway for the Dying Patient (LCP) on your ward or area, even if this patient is not within your group of patients for that shift. This should include ensuring that all parts of the LCP are completed appropriately, any variances are clearly documented and there is no missing data on the LCP. All LCPs are subject to regular audit, both locally and nationally.

- Be the key worker for the Continuous Quality Improvement Programme on your ward and you should ensure that you and your colleagues are aware of the relevant sections pertaining to end of life care on the Nursing Quality Performance Assessment Tool.

- Ensure that colleagues on your ward know where to access the LCP documents and supporting leaflets. You will take responsibility for regularly checking and organizing replenishment of the stock items in the LCP blue box file.

- Be expected to demonstrate that you have taken opportunities to raise awareness and carried out formal or informal teaching opportunities regarding end of life care with your colleagues; either on a 1:1 basis or in small groups. You will be expected to record any teaching carried out on your education personal record sheet (even if this has been a five minute session with one colleague, based on one goal of the LCP).

> **Box 9.1 As a Palliative Care Network Nurse at the Royal Liverpool and Broadgreen University Hospital NHS Trust you will** *(continued)*
>
> These record sheets will be collated at the end of each year by the HSPCT Lecturer Practitioner to monitor how this 'cascade model' of end of life care education is working.
>
> ♦ Be expected to take a lead role in educating ward colleagues regarding the safe use of the medical device that supports a continuous subcutaneous infusion and associated medicines management.
>
> ♦ Be expected to identify any difficulties or any additional support you need to carry out your ward based education to your line manager and to your nominated palliative care nurse specialist mentor at the earliest opportunity.
>
> ♦ In association with your line manager, you should be able to identify any staff from your area who would benefit from attending the (one day) HSPCT Foundation Day training in End of Life Care. You should ensure that they contact the HSPCT Lecturer Practitioner to allocate a date for this training.

Care of the dying is urgent care and must be seen as part of the core business of an organization; with training in end of life care, including care of the dying, as mandatory for all. A Network Nurse Programme can become an important part of the hospital framework for end of life care, alongside other important elements such as the inclusion of care of the dying at induction and mandatory training for all staff.

Evaluation and further training (Step 7)

Whilst ongoing reflection with the staff directly involved in the delivery of care using the LCP is of paramount importance, it is also useful to take the opportunity to reflect in a more formal, quantitative way once a sizeable amount of pathways have been used within the pilot sites. The LCP Central Team offers assistance to participating organizations to audit the first 20 LCPs used in the pilot site(s) in order to provide tangible feedback that can be disseminated more widely to key staff and highlight any improvements in the environment since the implementation of the LCP. The information gained from the audit can point to areas where further education or training would be useful and can lead to appropriate amendments to the ongoing education programme. It can also provide useful information about organizational issues, such as the availability (or otherwise) of resources, something that may need to be addressed in order to facilitate the delivery of high quality care.

The feedback report is of a similar format to that of the Base Review and, since the publication of version 12, has also been available in an electronic format that is immediately available to participating organizations when the data have been entered into the tool. The reports are designed to provide useful information in an accessible and easily interpretable format, using bar charts and tables to illustrate the proportion of 'achieved' (goal met), 'variance' (goal not met), and 'not required' codes on the LCP at the time of delivery of care, along with the proportion of missing data (ie nothing coded on the LCP against that particular goal).

Continuing development of competencies (Step 8)

Continuous development of the knowledge and skills of the workforce is necessary to embed the LCP model within the clinical environment to drive up quality in care of the dying.

Phase 4: Sustainability

Ongoing education, training, and support (Step 9); and the establishment of the LCP model within governance systems (Step 10)

These steps focus on the spread and sustainability of the LCP within a given organization. They involve the creation of structures and processes to underpin the continuing education required within the environment. Initiatives such as linking with local audit departments to encourage ongoing reflection on the quality of care delivery, keeping up to date with developments in end of life care, encouraging ongoing liaison with local specialist palliative care teams, participating in regional and national audits, and finding ways to represent end of life care within the governance and performance management structures of an organization, are all examples of the way that the LCP can become fully embedded within an organization.

Steps 8, 9, and 10 of the implementation programme are covered in more detail in Chapter 10.

Summary

The End of Life Care Strategy highlighted that although some people die as they would have wished, many do not (5). Many people still do not receive quality care at the end of their lives. In the past, the profile of end of life care across the NHS and across society has been relatively low, leading to variability in access to and the quality of end of life care across the country and in different communities.

The strategy acknowledges that there are many challenges to be overcome to ensure that everyone attains world class end of life care including care in the last hours or days of life, and this means that end of life care is now firmly established as an important aspect of healthcare delivery.

The LCP Continuous Quality Improvement Programme is recognized nationally and internationally as an effective means of improving end of life care. The programme incorporates change management techniques, education programmes, audit and research of demonstrable outcomes of care. When the LCP programme is implemented effectively it can help to ensure that everyone approaching the end of life has access to high quality care. This programme has the potential to change the culture of an organization to sustain the quality of care delivery at the bedside in the last hours or days of life.

References

1 Department of Health (2000). *NHS learning network: NHS beacon programme for 2000/2001*. DH.London.

2 Department of Health End of life care Programme (accessed 20 march 2010) http://www.endoflifecare.nhs.uk/eolc/

3 National Institute for Health and Clinical Excellence. *Improving supportive and palliative care for adults with cancer*. March 2004 (accessed 20 March 2010) http://www.nice.org.uk/csgsp

4 Department of Health. (2006) *Our health, our care, our say: a new direction for community services*, (accessed 20 March 2010).http://www.dh.gov.uk/en/Healthcare/Ourhealthourcareoursay/DH_065882

5 Department of Health (2008) *End of Life Care Strategy—promoting high quality care for all adults at the end of life*. DH. London

6 Department of Health (2009) *End of Life Care Strategy—Quality markers and measures for end of life care*. DH. London

7 National Care of the Dying Audit: *Hospitals summary reports* (2008/2009) accessed 20 March 2009 http://www.mcpcil.org.uk/pdfs/generic_NCDAH_2nd_Round_Final_Report%5B1%5D.pdf

8 Edwards-Deming W. (1994) *The new economics for industry, government, education*. 2nd ed. Massachusetts Institute of Technology Centre for Advanced Engineering Study.Massachusetts.

9 Hockley J, Dewar B, Watson J. Promoting end-of-life care in nursing homes using an 'integrated care pathway'. *J Res Nurs* 2005;**10**:135–52.

10 Mellor F, Foley T, Connolly M, Mercer V, Spanswick M. Role of a Clinical Facilitator in introducing an Integrated Care pathway for The Care Of The Dying. *Int J Palliat Nurs*, 2004;**10**(10):497–501.

11 Marie Curie Palliative Care Institute Liverpool, accessed 20 March 2010, http://www.mcpcil.org.uk/liverpool-care-pathway/documentation-lcp.htm#goaldata

12 Marie Curie Palliative Care Institute Liverpool, accessed 20 March 2010, http://www.mcpcil.org.uk/liverpool-care-pathway/documentation-lcp.htm

13 Graham, N. (ed) (1995) *Quality in health care: theory, application and evolution.* Aspen Publishers, Gaithersburg.

14 Schön D A. (1983) *The Reflective Practitioner: how professionals think in action.* Temple Smith, London.

15 National Statistics. Mortality Statistics. Series DH1 no. 38. Office for National Statistics, 2005. accessed 20 March 2010, http://www.statistics.gov.uk/downloads/theme_health/Dh1_38_2005/DH1_No_38.pdf

16 Jack B, Gambles M, Saltmarsh P, Murphy D, Hutchinson T, Ellershaw JE. Enhancing hospital nurses' knowledge of palliative care: a network nurse programme. *Int J Palliat Nurs,* 2004;**10**(10):502–6.

17 The Palliative Care Network Nurse Programme: Marie Curie Palliative care Institute Liverpool (MCPCIL) accessed 20 March 2010 http://www.mcpcil.org.uk/liverpool-care-pathway/learning-teaching.htm

Chapter 10

Dissemination and sustainability strategy for the LCP programme: incorporating a model for national audit for care of the dying

Deborah Murphy and Tamsin McGlinchey

The Liverpool Care Pathway for the Dying Patient (LCP) Continuous Quality Improvement Programme aims to achieve real and lasting improvements in the quality of care for patients in the last hours or days of life, for their relatives or carers, and for the health care professionals who support them. To implement, support, promote, and sustain quality within an organization there needs to be a clear understanding of what quality looks and feels like with an understanding of measurement to drive improvement. Quality is defined in different ways by different organizations. In general terms good quality care should be safe, effective, patient centred, timely, efficient, equitable, and measurable. It should deliver value for money and will be provided within a broader framework of health care performance within a system that has the capacity to drive and respond to this agenda.

Appropriate and timely information regarding quality of care will assist clinical systems, providers, and commissioners to improve services and make it easier to share best practice so that organizations remain productive by continually learning and innovating. The measurement of quality to drive up improvement is without doubt a requirement of a high performing healthcare system. If the benefits of quality measurement are to have maximum impact on the care provided in the last hours or days of life then an organization will need to articulate measures that meet the needs of diverse stakeholders, patients, carers, providers, and commissioners. There will need to be a system to compare information across the health economy within a regulatory framework of governance and risk and a willingness to share best practice in support of continual development.

Clinical governance in this respect is essentially an organizational concept aimed at ensuring that every heath organization creates the culture, systems, and support mechanisms so that good clinical performance supporting care in the last hours or days of life will be the norm. Continuous quality improvement in care of the dying will therefore become part and parcel of routine clinical practice wherever patients die.

The LCP however is only as good as the teams that are using it. The implementation and dissemination of the LCP into an organization will create a change process in the environment. However change is organized, there is a need to ensure the capacity and capability in terms of people with the right skills, knowledge, attitude, and support to properly enable the scale and pace of the change required.

Recognition of the fundamental aspects of a change management programme is pivotal to success when implementing and disseminating the LCP. The Service Improvement Model used at the Marie Curie Palliative Care Institute Liverpool (MCPCIL) is a four-phased approach incorporating a 10 step continuous quality improvement process for the LCP Programme (see Chapter 2). Steps 9 and 10 within this process focus on the spread and sustainability of the LCP within a given organization. They involve the creation of structures and processes to underpin the continuing education required within the environment. Initiatives such as linking with local audit departments to encourage ongoing reflection on the quality of care delivery; keeping up to date with developments in end of life care; encouraging ongoing liaison with local specialist palliative care teams; participating in regional and national audits; and finding ways to represent end of life care within the governance and performance management structures of an organization; are all examples of the way that the LCP can become fully embedded within an organization.

Sustainable healthcare systems are created when clinical leaders are empowered to bring about transformational change supported by managers who back good ideas or best practice models like the LCP, remove blockages to progress, and provide consistent support. Whilst the LCP Central Team plays an enabling role in this change process the real changes will be designed, delivered, measured, and sustained locally.

The structure of the LCP makes it potentially easy to audit and provide ongoing, relevant, and up to date information concerning aspects of care delivery in the dying phase. It also enables comparative audit with other organizations that are using the LCP document. Data can be brought together to illustrate care in a wider context and to allow organizations to understand their own level of comparative audit in relation to similar settings. This opportunity to reflect on one's own performance in comparison with that of others locally, regionally or nationally is invaluable in promoting continuous quality improvement in care of the dying.

National clinical audit in context

Since the 1989 White Paper *Working For Patients* (1), the use of national clinical audit has been a key part of Clinical Governance, to monitor and evaluate clinical services within the NHS. National clinical audit involves the frequent review of the delivery of healthcare services, to ensure that best practice is being carried out. A recent definition of national clinical audit is a 'quality improvement process that seeks to improve patient care and outcomes through systematic review of care against explicit criteria' (NICE, 2002) (2). Good clinical audit will identify problems and effect changes that result in improved outcomes in patient care.

A review by CAPSE (3,4) highlighted that the interface between national audit through to local audit and evaluation was in need of review. The report proposed that the medical colleges had the potential to lead clinical audits and develop 'comparative analyses' to further develop the impact of national clinical audit on local audit and the development of policies and procedures. In 1997 the Healthcare Executive commissioned the National Sentinel Audits, conducted in collaboration with various medical colleges, in order to develop the role of clinical audit as a means to improve quality of care delivery. National clinical audit has been widely used in the NHS to monitor the provision of healthcare, and its importance in 'driving up' the quality of healthcare provided in the UK has been demonstrated through the development of National Guidelines (through the National Institute for Clinical Excellence) to promote 'best practice' in healthcare provision. More recently, it has been said that national audit has 'lacked a national strategy and a coherent programme of activities' (5) and so to reinvigorate and improve how national audit is delivered, the Department of Health set up the National Clinical Audit Advisory Group (NCAAG) in 2008 (5). The principal purpose of NCAAG is to improve and increase the impact of clinical audit, as a means to support local and national improvements to clinical practice and service delivery.

The impact of national clinical audit

Ongoing monitoring and evaluation of the healthcare system in the UK has been moving in the direction of 'NHS Targets' and 'Quality Markers'(6), in order that individual organizations can measure themselves against determined 'national standards', that are then fed into the Trust Board/Management agenda through the local Clinical Governance framework in order to identify locally any areas for improvement, and to aid commissioners in the funding of services.

National clinical audit has become an effective tool, for monitoring and promoting change within individual organizations, when employed within a Continuous Quality Improvement Programme (CQIP) (7). This process facilitates audit against 'national standards', by comparing performance across different organizations against those standards, and promoting the development of local action plans in order to effect change in the local healthcare environment. This utility of benchmarking allows organizations to reflect on their own performance at a local level, in relation to the national picture, allowing a more meaningful dissemination of the audit findings, and creating an 'audit cycle', enabling an iterative approach to change. Lilford et al. (8) describe this as an 'examination of existing processes, change, monitoring the apparent effects of the change, and further change'.

An example of this continuous quality improvement process can be seen in the National Sentinel Audit in Stroke conducted by the Intercollegiate Working Party for Stroke, coordinated by the Clinical Effectiveness and Evaluations Unit (CEEU) at the Royal College of Physicians (9). Evidence suggests that well organized care of patients with stroke, on a designated stroke unit has clear associations with decreased mortality and longer term conditions. In the first round of the audit on average 19% of patients received most of their care on a designated stoke unit; but after extensive dissemination of the results, individual action planning for improvements in care delivery, and time to implement any changes necessary, the results from the second round showed that this had increased to 26% (in Trusts who took part in both rounds). Analysis of the 'change questionnaire' indicated that 31 new stroke units opened between the first and second rounds of the audit.

This standardized approach to audit, benchmarking, and comprehensive dissemination is invaluable, and it is recognized as a crucial part in the continuous improvement of services provided by the health care system (HQIP, 2010) (10). It has been recommended that all providers of healthcare should participate in comparative clinical audit and use the results to support local and national clinical governance (DH, 2004) (11). All NHS Trusts are currently monitored by the Care Quality Commission (CQC), previously the Healthcare Commission (HC), and Trusts wishing to register with the CQC will have to provide evidence that clinical audit work is being carried out.

The next section describes how the LCP, as part of a Continuous Quality Improvement Programme, can be used for audit and evaluation at a national level. This is demonstrated through the National Care of the Dying Audit—Hospitals (NCDAH). This national audit used aggregated data to provide

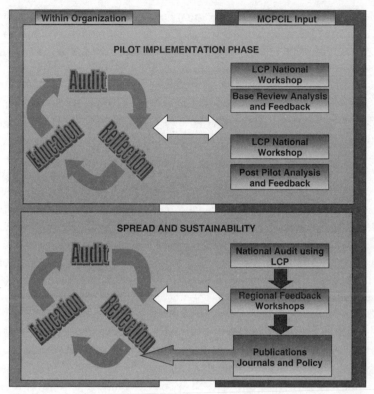

Fig. 10.1 The cycle of continuous audit, reflection, and education and training Taken from 'Continuous quality improvement in care of the dying with the Liverpool Care Pathway for the Dying Patient' (2009) (12).

a 'National Benchmark' of care of the dying in hospitals that is used both nationally to create a 'picture' of care in the last hours or days of life, and locally to compare performance across similar organizations. The audit enables the management of an organization to drive up quality of care for dying patients from the executive board to the bedside. Critical reflection on current clinical practice around care of the dying is also promoted which enables education and training to be focused appropriately to improve care. Figure 10.1 gives a visual representation of the cycle of continuous audit, reflection, and education and training.

NCDAH: driving up quality in care of the dying as part of a Continuous Quality Improvement Programme

The Marie Curie Palliative Care Institute Liverpool (MCPCIL), in collaboration with the Royal College of Physicians and supported by the Department of Health End of Life Care Programme (13) and Marie Curie Cancer Care, have undertaken two rounds of the National Care of the Dying Audit Hospitals (NCDAH), with data collection for round one in autumn 2006 (14), and round two in autumn 2008 (15). The primary aims of both rounds of the NCDAH were to enable participating hospitals to identify the quality of their care for dying patients as documented on the LCP; and to allow them to compare their performance with other participating hospitals; and action plan for future care delivery. The full generic reports for both rounds of the NCDAH can be found on the MCPCIL website (*www.mcpcil.org.uk*).

The Department of Health 'quality markers' for end of life care (6) have included 'the submission of data into local and national audits of care of the dying' as one of the top 10 markers of quality for organizations caring for dying patients. It is intended that the NCDAH will be repeated on a two yearly cycle, giving hospitals the opportunity to report back nationally relevant data regarding care delivered to patients supported by the LCP to their Trust Board, by positioning themselves against the 'national benchmark'. This supports hospitals to spotlight areas for improvement, but also to celebrate success where performance in the audit has been identified as good.

Method and audit sample

A retrospective audit design was used to gather data relevant to each of the goals of care on the LCP from up to 30 consecutive deaths in each of the participating hospitals over a three month period (Round 1: data from 118 hospitals and 2672 patients; Round 2: data from 155 hospitals and 3893 patients). Round 2 of the NCDAH included data from 82% of all relevant NHS Trusts in England. Pertinent patient and hospital organizational data were also gathered to contextualize the data from the LCP and to aid interpretation of the results. Data were primarily analysed using descriptive statistics and participating hospitals received a report illustrating their own performance against the aggregate performance for all patients.

For both round 1 and round 2, in order to start to close the 'audit loop' in the CQIP process, a maximum of three representatives from each hospital took part in one of three regional workshops. These regional workshops took place between three and six months after publication of the reports to allow participants time to reflect on their own results prior to the workshops. These workshops gave participating staff the opportunity to revisit the findings; network with others; identify barriers and review education and training in care of the dying; and to begin the process of action planning for future improvement. Participants were asked to complete an exit questionnaire about the perceived value of reports, the workshops, and participation in the audit.

Most questions required participants to rate their agreement with a series of statements on a five-point scale from strongly agree to strongly disagree.

Findings from the National Care of the Dying Audit—Hospitals (NCDAH)

The results presented in this chapter are taken from the NCDAH Round 2 report, and are presented as an example of the type of information that participating hospitals received. These results are used to show how the use of objective data can offer important insights on several levels. Firstly, at individual hospital level, it is possible to compare one's own performance with that of other similar organizations, to identify where performance falls below the standard of others, and therefore, where future education and training should be focused. Secondly, they illustrate at a national level which goals of care are routinely achieved for patients in the dying phase, as well as those goals where improvement is required, providing the opportunity to feed into national policy in terms of standards and guidelines around care of the dying.

The results were presented in a simple format to allow easy interpretation. They were displayed in tables showing individual hospital performance against the 'national benchmark', and also illustrating (for those hospitals that provided at least 10 patient data sets) hospital variation in performance on goals of care on the LCP in the form of box plots. These box plots allowed individual hospitals to position themselves in the top 25%, middle 50%, or bottom 25% (the 'inter-quartile range') of participating hospitals, although hospital identity was confidential.

Figure 10.2 illustrates the tables, presenting individual hospital performance (represented in 'Your Site') against the 'national benchmark' (represented in 'NCDAH Round 2'). Importantly in these tables, as well as the percentage of times a goal was documented as 'achieved', individual hospitals were able to identify the proportion of times a goal was documented as a 'variance', and also the proportion of times that a goal was 'not documented' at the point of care delivery.

Figures 10.3, 10.4, and 10.5 illustrate the box plots displayed to show hospital variation. They illustrate the spread of hospitals with the highest and lowest values for each goal (not defined as outliers), shown by the 'whiskers' above and below the green boxes. The green boxes themselves illustrate the percentage of 'achieved' for the middle 50% of hospitals and the median value is represented by the thick black line within each box. An 'outlier' is represented by a 'circle' highlighting those hospitals whose percentage 'achieved' falls more than one and a half 'box lengths' above or below the green box. An 'extreme outlier' is represented by a 'star' highlighting those hospitals whose percentage

LCP Goal 1: Current medication assessed and non-essentials discontinued

	Available & Applicable	Achieved		Variance		Not documented	
	N	%	N	%	N	%	N
Your Site Round 2	30	97	29	0	-	3	1
National Round 2	3864	92	3547	1	47	7	270
Hospital IQR – all (%) (n = 153)		87 – 97%		0 – 3%		0 – 10%	
National Round 1	2633	93	2442	2	55	5	136

LCP Goal 2: PRN subcutaneous medication written up for list below as per protocol

	Available & Applicable	Achieved		Variance		Not documented	
	N	%	N	%	N	%	N
2.1 Pain							
Your Site Round 2	30	93	28	3	1	3	1
National Round 2	3863	90	3476	3	128	7	259
Hospital IQR - all (%) (n=154)		87 – 97%		0 – 3%		0 – 10%	
National Round 1	2671	91	2418	4	95	6	158

Fig. 10.2 Example of individual hospital feedback showing the results for goals 1 and 2.1 (LCP generic version 11) from Round 2 of the NCDAH. Aggregated data shown is accurate; data represented in 'Your Site' is for example purposes only. NCDAH Round 2.

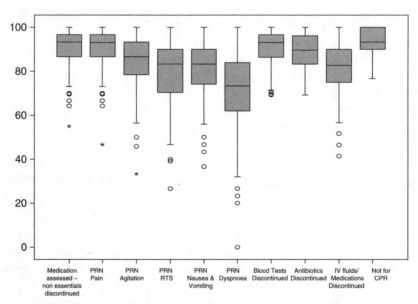

Fig. 10.3 Domain 1 box plot: physical comfort of the patient (initial assessment). Box plots include only hospitals that were able to provide 10 or more patient data sets.

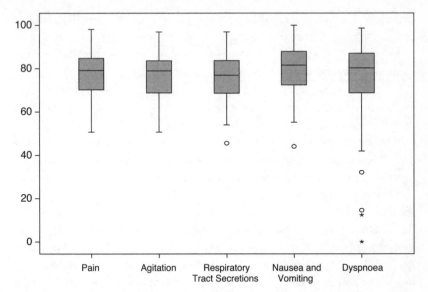

Fig. 10.4 Domain 1 box plot: physical comfort of the patient (ongoing assessment). Box plots include only hospitals that were able to provide 10 or more patient data sets.

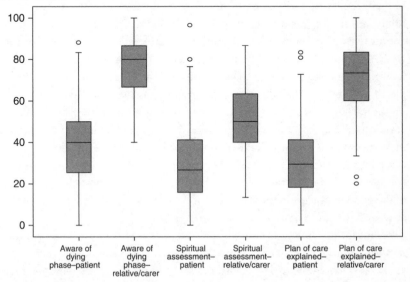

Fig. 10.5 Domains 2 and 3: psychological and spiritual/religious aspects of care and communication.

'achieved' falls three box lengths above or below the green box. The value of presenting the results to individual hospitals in this way is so they can flag up areas for scrutiny, where others have performed well, and prompt the development of a local action plan to effect change for improvement into the future.

Nationally, these results can illustrate important variations in the overall level of performance for different goals of care and between hospitals in the sample. Figures 10.3, 10.4, and 10.5 also illustrate these differences.

In the last hours or days of life, ensuring patient comfort is the main focus of care once the decision has been made that a patient is unlikely to survive the current episode of care. Having medications prescribed for the most commonly occurring symptoms so that they are available should they be required is an important element in the drive to ensure patient comfort. The results from the NCDAH Round 2 illustrate that for the majority of patients and within the majority of hospitals, these medications have been prescribed appropriately (Figure 10.3). Similarly, when looking at the ongoing assessment of the condition of the patient as documented in the four hourly assessments over the last 24 hours of life, patients were found to be comfortable in terms of these symptoms (Figure 10.4). In the main, this information provides important positive outcomes for patients in the last hours or days of life, but also, those hospitals that identify themselves as 'outliers' can also pinpoint areas for improvement.

Some interesting variations in the level of documentation at the end of life are also worthy of note, for example, the relatively greater variation apparent in the level of discontinuation of intravenous fluids/medications. This is an important finding, as it may reflect individual clinician decision-making to continue with such interventions in the best interest of the patient. For the NCDAH Round 2, the documented reasons for the continuation of intravenous fluids/medications were collected, although it was relatively poorly completed, with only 17% of documented variances having a corresponding entry on the variance sheet. This has the potential to provide richer information around this goal, and variances that were documented highlighted that in the most cases it was the medical decision to continue for reasons such as: continue current IV fluid bag then stop; continue fluids until cannula tissues; continue for 24 hours and review. This is invaluable when providing a picture of the patient journey in the last hours or days of life, although better compliance with variance recording is imperative.

Results for psychological and spiritual/religious aspects of care and communication around the plan of care, particularly with the patient, illustrate larger variation across individual hospitals, and much lower levels of achievement for these goals of care (Figure 10.5). Some areas of good practice are identified however, with some hospitals achieving 100% for these goals, meaning that there is the potential for improvement in order to raise that national standard, by reflecting on and using these results to open up the debate within and between hospitals to identify education and training needs. Again in the NCDAH Round 2, variances documented on the variance sheet were collected for religious and spiritual needs of the relatives or carers, however, this was also relatively poorly completed, with only 19% of variances backed up with written information on the variance sheet.

Key performance indicators (KPIs)

A series of key performance indicators were developed for the first time in the second round of the NCDAH to provide an 'at a glance' picture of performance against some of the key elements in the delivery of care to dying patients and their relatives or carers. These indicators were developed in order to be usefully included on the 'corporate performance dashboard' used in many Trusts to promote continuous quality improvement, and to raise the profile of care of the dying, and the use of the LCP. The KPIs are data driven benchmarks that focus on the following issues:

- ◆ Key performance indicator 1: Spread of the LCP
- ◆ Key performance indicator 2: Anticipatory prescribing for the key symptoms that may develop in the last hours or days of life
- ◆ Key performance indicator 3: Compliance with completion of the LCP or equivalent pathway.

One of the recommendations from the NCDAH Round 2 Generic Report was that 'Key Performance Indicators (KPIs) for care of the dying should be measured, monitored, and managed as part of the organization 'corporate performance dashboard'. This is one way that care of the dying can be brought into the mainstream monitoring of the organization, providing a mechanism for regular performance review. Figure 10.6 provides an example of KPI 2. Box 10.1 outlines the 10 recommendations from this round of the national audit.

Anticipatory prescribing for key symptoms	Your Site Round 2 (n=30)	National Round 2 (n=101)
Median % (IQR)	91%	88% (83%–94%)
0% – 82%	83% – 94%	95% – 100%

Fig. 10.6 Example of 'Key Performance Indicator' provided within the NCDAH Round 2. Key performance indicator 2: anticipatory prescribing for the key symptoms that may develop in the last hours or days of life.

Box 10.1 NCDAH Round 2 Key Recommendations (2009)

1. Key Performance Indicators (KPIs) for care of the dying should be measured, monitored, and managed as part of the organization corporate performance dashboard.

2. All hospitals should have a clear programme for continuous quality improvement for care of the dying to drive up performance and quality. A remedial action plan in response to National Care of the Dying Audit findings should be in place to address poor compliance, inter-quartile range (IQR) outliers, variance reporting, and improved performance across the key domains of care.

3. A named person within the organization should take formal responsibility to act as an LCP Facilitator/change agent for care of the dying.

4. Whilst the median doses prescribed and given for agitation and restlessness (both prn and continuous subcutaneous infusion) are relatively low, audit sites that are frequently prescribing outside the 90th percentile need to review practice. Audit sites where morphine and diamorphine have been prescribed for this symptom should also review their practice.

5. All hospitals should have a local audit programme for care of the dying that includes the assessment of the views of bereaved carers.

6. Optimizing knowledge transfer is an important aspect of continuous quality improvement. All hospitals should have appropriate information leaflets available in support of care in the last hours or days of life.

7. Hospitals need to identify the reasons for the relatively poorer performance on goals that deal with patient insight (both into diagnosis and recognition of dying) and spiritual assessment (for both patients and carers). All health care workers caring for dying patients and their relatives or carers should have access to appropriate ongoing training and education in care of the dying (DH 2009).

8. The use of the Care After Death Section of the LCP for all deaths has been recommended (DH 2009). This audit shows that there is a high proportion of missing data for all goals in the Care After Death Section and it is therefore important that hospitals identify the reasons for this.

> **Box 10.1 NCDAH Round 2 Key Recommendations (2009)** *(continued)*
>
> 9. The Department of Health's Quality Markers and Measures for End of Life Care (DH 2009) document recommends that all hospitals take part in the two yearly National Care of the Dying Audit Cycle.
> 10. All hospitals should have an LCP or equivalent in place (DH 2009) that is compliant with the goals included in the new updated version 12 of the LCP, published in November 2009.

Workshop outcomes

Participation in the workshops, 3–6 months after the publication of the report, encouraged further reflection on the results and was positively evaluated. Further reflection and discussion of the results of the audit allowed individuals to 'tease' out the issues underlying performance for their individual hospital and to share areas of current good practice in response to these issues. Participants were asked to identify on 'sticky boards' any education and training initiatives for care of the dying that were currently being utilized in their organization. These initiatives were then themed on the spot by the workshop facilitators, and individuals were encouraged to peruse these education and training initiatives in order to start the process of 'networking' with others to improve and develop education in their own organization.

The main issues identified included raising the importance of good education and training in end of life care both locally and nationally, embedding it within already existing structures such as the Trust mandatory training system for local education and training, and nationally for and pre registration nursing and medical students. The importance of having an LCP facilitator in the environment to identify education and training needs, and to facilitate delivery of that education, was highlighted as a key requirement for the continued use and sustainability of the LCP within individual hospitals. Mandatory training in care of the dying was a key request from participants in support of sustainable best practice.

The process of action planning for the future began as part of the workshop process to identify the areas that need most attention in order to keep the use and sustainability of the LCP at an optimum level. Set in a broader strategy for continuous quality improvement an action planning process can ensure that the outputs and learning are transformed into action and appropriate effective change.

LCP version 12 consultation exercise

Following the publication of the results of the first round of the NCDAH in November 2007 a two year consultation exercise was undertaken regarding the LCP generic version 11 document. The aim was to consult on potential changes to the content and design of the existing document as part of the Continuous Quality Improvement Programme to create LCP generic version 12. There was an opportunity to capture experience, attitude, and opinion from a wide range of activities across the UK and from international colleagues. This included feedback from both national audits, the experience of relatives and carers, healthcare professionals, and national organizations.

The exercise was extensive and the response from all stakeholders was excellent. Relatives and carers talked about the moments of engagement between them and health care professionals and the emotions and memories that these moments created. The need for compassion, dignity and respect, and written information to underpin any complex or sensitive conversation was highlighted. Relatives and carers spoke of the need to be included in all decision making processes as active participants in this process, not just being informed of a decision or situation or have euphemistic language used.

The ethos of the LCP generic document has remained unchanged. LCP version 12 has greater clarity in key areas particularly communication, nutrition, and hydration. Care of the dying patient and their relative or carer can be supported effectively by the version 11 or 12 LCP document. Box 10.2 shows examples within the LCP generic version 12 where goals of care are more specifically articulated. A full copy of the LCP core documentation can be viewed in Appendix 1.

Summary

Measurement of quality to drive sustained improvement is pivotal for a high-performing healthcare system, and the national and international focus on measurement and quality indicators for care of the dying is likely to continue. However, for this initiative to achieve its potential all organizations need to be able to respond to the opportunities and challenges that it presents.

Data can be a powerful tool for improving quality of care. Effective use of measurement tools must be an essential part of strategic growth within an organization and reflected within a governance and risk portfolio. The LCP programme supports clinicians to provide best quality care in the last hours or days of life. As an integrated care pathway it can be used to audit documentation and care delivery, and to benchmark between similar organizations. The LCP used within a National Care of the Dying Audit is a major lever to improve care of the dying.

Box 10.2 Examples within the LCP generic version 12 where goals of care are more specifically articulated

- Multidisciplinary Team (MDT) Decision Making

  The recognition and diagnosis of dying is always complex: uncertainty is an integral part of dying. There are occasions when a patient thought to be dying lives longer than expected and vice versa. Seek a second opinion or specialist palliative care support as needed. The decision that a patient is thought to be dying and the LCP commenced to support the care in the last hours or days of life requires the senior clinician ultimately responsible for the patient's care to document this decision. LCP generic version 12—UK contains a helpful algorithm to support clinical decision making

- Communication

  Good communication is pivotal to best quality of care in the last hours or days of life—LCP generic version 12 has a front 'tear off' sheet for you to give to a relative or carer to reflect your conversation with the patient, where possible and deemed appropriate, and the relative or carer. The views of all concerned must be listened to and documented.

- Formal MDT review every 3 days

  The LCP includes ongoing review of the needs of the patient and the relative or carer. The patient will need to be formally reviewed every 3 days by the MDT to ensure that all clinicians, the patient where possible, and the relative or carer are in agreement with current decisions and if consensus cannot be reached support from a second opinion or the palliative care team can be sought.

  A review of the current plan of care should also be triggered if one or more of the following apply:

  > Improved conscious level, functional ability, oral intake, mobility, ability to perform self care
  > Concerns expressed regarding the management plan by the patient, relative or carer, or team member
  > It is three days since the last full MDT assessment

- Review of the need for clinically assisted nutrition or hydration:

  Goals 6, 7 and K—The need for clinically assisted nutrition or hydration (CANH) is reviewed by the MDT. The LCP does not preclude the use of CANH. All clinical decisions must be made in the patient's best interest

- Assess the patient's skin integrity—goal 8:

  The aim is to prevent pressure ulcers or further deterioration if a pressure ulcer is present

The LCP is not the answer to the challenges for caring for dying patients and their relatives and carers in our society but is a step in the right direction. It is imperative to amplify the voice of patients where possible and relatives and carers as drivers of service delivery and innovation. Rigorous evaluation of the impact of the LCP is required by international experience to continue in the development and application of quality measures for care in the last hours or days of life.

References

1 Department of Health (1989) *Working for Patients*. Department of Health. London: HMSO.

2 National Institute for Clinical Excellence (2002) *Principles for Best Practice in Clinical Audit*. Abingdon, Oxon: Radcliffe Medical Press.

3 Amess M, Walshe K, Shaw C, Coles J (1995) *Evaluating Audit Activities of the Medical Royal Colleges and Their Faculties in England*. CAPSE Research, London.

4 Wilmott M, Foster J, Walshe K, and Coles J (1995) *Evaluating Audit: A Review of Audit Activity in the Nursing and Therapy Professions: Findings of a National Survey*. CAPSE Research, London.

5 National Clinical Audit Advisory Group (NCAG) http://www.dh.gov.uk/ab/NCAAG/index.htm (accessed 20 April 2010).

6 Department of Health (2009) *End of life Care Strategy: quality markers and measures for end of life care*. Department of Health, London.

7 Rudd A G, Lowe D, Irwin P, Rutledge Z, Pearson M. National stroke audit: a tool for change? *Qual Health Care*, 2001;**10**:141–51.

8 Lilford R, Warren R, Braunholtz D. Action research: a way of researching or a way of managing? *J Health Serv Res Policy* 2003;**8**:100–4.

9 Clinical Effectiveness and Evaluations Unit (CEEU), Royal College of Physicians (RCP). *National Sentinel Audit of Stroke*. http://www.rcplondon.ac.uk/clinical-standards/ceeu/Completed-work/Pages/Stroke-audit.aspx (accessed 20 April 2010).

10 Healthcare Quality Improvement Partnership (HQIP) (2010) *Clinical Audit: A Simple Guide for NHS Boards and Partners*, HQIP, London.

11 Department of Health (2004) *National Standards, Local Action: Health and Social Care Standards and Planning Framework 2005/06–2007/08*. Department of Health, London.

12 Gambles M, McGlinchey T, Aldridge J, Murphy D, Ellershaw J. Continuous quality improvement in care of the dying with the Liverpool Care Pathway for the Dying Patient. International *J Care Pathw*, 2009;**13**:51–56.

13 Department of Health (2008) *End of Life Care Strategy: Promoting High Quality Care for all Adults at the End of Life*. Department of Health, London.

14 Marie Curie Palliative Care Institute Liverpool (2007) *National Care of the Dying Audit Hospitals: Round 1 Generic Report*, via http://www.mcpcil.org.uk/liverpool-care-path-way/pdfs/NCDAHGENERICREPORTFINAL-Auglockedpdf.pdf (accessed 16 April 2010).

15 Marie Curie Palliative Care Institute Liverpool (2009) *National Care of the Dying Audit Hospitals: Round 2 Generic Report*, via http://www.mcpcil.org.uk/pdfs/Generic_NCDAH_2nd_Round_Final_Report%5B1%5D.pdf (accessed 16 April 2010).

Chapter 11

International development of the Liverpool Care Pathway for the Dying Patient (LCP)

Ruthmarijke Smeding, Maria Bolger, and John Ellershaw

LCP International: setting the scene

The modern hospice movement was introduced by Cicely Saunders with the opening of St Christopher's Hospice in London in 1967. Palliative medicine is considered a young discipline within medicine with continuing debate regarding its terminology and shared standards. Following this pioneering stage of the specialty, that Ferris et al. refer to as 'the grass roots movement developed where there were champions' (1), there has been a consistent momentum to improve the quality of care for all those with advanced incurable life limiting disease including care of the dying and into bereavement. However, measurement and comparison of service provision and outcomes across communities remains challenging. The European Association for Palliative Care (EAPC) has recently recommended advocating standards and norms to further support stakeholder awareness about hospice and palliative care in Europe and determine a more appropriate equitable service delivery (2).

The World Health Organization (WHO) strongly advises policy-makers to ensure that palliative care is integral to the work of all healthcare services and is not seen as an additional extra (3). The Council of Europe recommends that national healthcare strategies should include measures for the development and functional integration of palliative care (4).

Integrated Care Pathways (ICP) as outlined in Chapter 1 are a clear means to determine best practice for a well defined group of patients during a well defined period. The Liverpool Care Pathway for the Dying Patient (LCP) is an example of an ICP that can determine best evidence based practice for those in the last hours or days of life. In the UK with its established specialty of palliative medicine it is absolutely reasonable to suggest that although the LCP is a generic document it should be implemented and supported by specialist palliative care. However, for many international colleagues in situations where palliative care is not as well established and standards and norms are not as well articulated the LCP has indeed been implemented but has always required strong consistent leadership. It is important to remember that the best quality of LCP implementation is dependant on equitable access to support, and learning and teaching. The capability for research and innovation and international benchmarking in care of the dying is dependant on a number of key considerations;

An agreed audit tool—e.g. the LCP

Maintaining the integrity of the LCP

International cultural norms

International policy, procedure, and legislation

Clinical governance and risk frameworks.

It is not perhaps the similarity of palliative care services across states or countries that makes this possible, but the shared dedication and need for change to provide all of us with a dignified death.

LCP international activity

Since 2000 the LCP Central Team at the Marie Curie Palliative Care Institute Liverpool (MCPCIL) has been working with a number of palliative care and oncology leads in several countries around the world regarding the development, implementation, and dissemination of the LCP programme. As described above, there was on the one hand the UK with its well established palliative care approach, and on the other hand, many countries where palliative care was in its infancy with new structures for palliative care integration being developed within their healthcare systems. This has led over time to a mutual learning of how best to integrate the LCP programme in other countries. Based on evaluation of this learning an LCP International Programme has developed. As with the UK LCP Continuous Quality Improvement Programme (CQIP) (see Chapter 9) the LCP International Programme includes a four-phased change management process (see Chapter 2, Table 2.1). This process clarifies issues including governance and risk, intellectual property, and ongoing research and development collaborations.

Each phase includes work streams to reflect clinical expertise and decision making; management and leadership; learning and teaching; research and development, including metrics and measurement; and governance and risk (see Figure 11.1).

To maintain the integrity of the LCP programme it is important to collaborate with colleagues within English and non English speaking countries. Learning in support of a continuous quality improvement process, and the development of the research and innovation agenda for care of the dying will be enhanced if it is agreed that the goals on the core LCP model remain unchanged. This process will also support future potential benchmarking models. The international LCP registered activity with the LCP Central Team is demonstrated within 3 levels. These levels apply to a state or country and will include a degree of contractual obligation.

Level 1 (State / Country)
When any organization / institution within a state or a country is registered with the LCP Central Team. This activity is driven by each individual organization independently and is not coordinated by a designated state or country lead.

Level 2 (State / Country)
When any organization / institution across a state or country is registered with the LCP Central Team and there is a recognized LCP lead who coordinates the LCP activity across a region or geographical location.

Level 3 (State / Country)
When the state / country has achieved national endorsement and funding within the state / country's health care system for the LCP programme. There will be a state / country nominated lead and a recognized LCP office with a full legally binding agreement in place with the LCP Central Team.

Throughout this chapter there are examples in practice of the challenges, opportunities and experiences of implementation of the LCP from an international perspective.

Phase 1: Induction—establishing the project and preparing the environment for organizational change

This phase is the most intensive and may take months to complete. Implementation of the LCP requires a 'top down, bottom up' approach to ensure all stakeholders agree the main aim which is to improve care in the last hours or days of life. A major cultural shift across an organization is required if the needs of dying patients are to be met and the workforce are to be empowered to take a leading role in this process.

The organization will need to register with the LCP Central Team. This involves completion of an electronic registration form and uploading a letter of endorsement from the chief executive/manager of the organization.

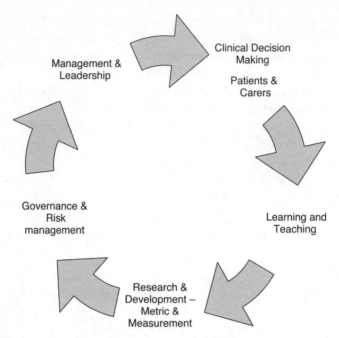

Fig. 11.1 5 key work streams representing organizational governance.

Executive/senior management support within the organization is essential for the success of implementing the LCP. A small group of enthusiastic individuals will not create a sustainable project into the future unless executive teams are fully able to endorse the LCP programme. The LCP logo, referencing of documents, and other elements of intellectual property and copyright issues need to be agreed.

Leadership and establishing a steering group

A local steering group is essential to take the project forward. This group needs to be driven by a lead, usually a clinician who has some understanding of the LCP programme. The lead should be able to implement the LCP model as a pilot phase within his or her clinical area and drive the LCP agenda forward.

At the initial steering group meeting it is important to discuss with the stakeholders the aims of the LCP programme:

- ◆ To empower generic workers
- ◆ To improve care for the dying patient
- ◆ To demonstrate outcomes of care for dying patients
- ◆ To improve the experience of relatives or carers in relation to care of the dying, grief, and bereavement

◆ To determine that care of the dying is part of the core business of the organization

◆ To promote care of the dying as a quality indicator across the organization

A full understanding of the LCP will be required—the LCP Central Team can support learning in this area with ongoing telephone contact, learning materials, and email support.

◆ Recognition and diagnosis of dying

◆ Layout of the document—importance of goals and outcomes

Section 1: Initial assessment

Section 2: Ongoing assessment

Section 3: Care after death

◆ It is important to understand the LCP is a multi-professional document

◆ It is important to understand the importance of variance (see Chapter 2 for a full explanation).

The project should where possible be endorsed and supported by an academic institution/university. The project proposal and aims need to be written up and sent to the LCP Central Team. Appropriate administrative support is important to the success of the project.

Translation

If the LCP is to be used in a language other than English then a translation process following EORTC guidelines should be completed (5). The LCP Central Team must endorse the final translated LCP document before it can be used in clinical practice. Any supportive literature/leaflets that carry the LCP logo must be reviewed by the LCP Central Team.

Learning and teaching

This programme will only be successful if fully supported by a robust and continuous education and training programme. There is some material and support available from the LCP Central Team, but much depends on the needs of the environment and must be locally driven. This is resource intensive at the outset and needs to be a realistic teaching programme that can be sustained. A key change agent in the environment is needed, although the scope of this role should change over time. The LCP Central Team suggests an LCP facilitator approach. The LCP facilitator will need to familiarize themselves with the 10 Step Continuous Quality Improvement Programme (see Chapter 9).

Testing the change ideas

The LCP Central Team recommends consideration of the use of the PDSA cycle (Deming 1994) as part of the model for improvement (6). This enables the implementation of the LCP into a pilot site and to learn from its potential impact. This is quite different from the approach traditionally used in health-care settings.

There are four stages to the cycle:

+ **Plan:** agree the change to be implemented
+ **Do:** carry out the change and measure the impact
+ **Study:** study data before and after the change and reflect on learning
+ **Act:** Plan the next change cycle or implementation

This PDSA cycle supports the key questions:

+ What are we trying to achieve?
+ How will we know if the change is an improvement?
+ What changes can we make that will sustain the improvements we seek?

Research and development

The steering group will need to consider what success looks like and how to measure improvement. A reflective process will need to be adopted. Success will be more than just the number of LCPs used in the environment. Successful change may be demonstrated in any number of ways, change in knowledge, skill, or attitude of clinical teams. Clinical teams may have increased confidence and competence to care for patients and support their relatives in the dying phase. There may be a change to the physical environment and associated facilities available. Innovation and change may be demonstrated by enhanced communication or more open shared ways of learning or working.

Some areas have been able to create a more demonstrable evidence base for the LCP or demonstrate enhanced symptom control. Some organizations have used the initial learning from the LCP programme as a means to collate a more robust research proposal to examine more complex issues such as diagnosing dying.

Governance and risk

The steering group will need to take ownership of the governance and risk agenda for this project. The LCP is only as good as the teams using it and the group will need to take responsibility for the ongoing future development of this programme and ensure it reflects best governance both in clinical, business, and quality assurance. All potential changes to the current LCP document must be agreed with the LCP Central Team. Current LCP goals of care must remain unchanged; if you feel that the goals do not reflect your practice we suggest charting this as a variance. This enables us to build together evidence for the cultural, traditional, and structural differences between countries for good care of the dying. It is possible to have additional goals on the LCP to address specific organizational policy or cultural needs.

International perspective

LCP in Argentina: time to build the bases to make a difference

Despite a relatively steady expansion during the last 10 years, palliative care services in Argentina are still quite scarce and don't reach the vast majority of patients who might benefit from them. This fact encouraged us to optimize research and education for the care of cancer and non cancer patients in the last days of life. We found the Liverpool Care Pathway for the Dying Patient (LCP) to be a proper instrument to guide and enable health care professionals to focus on care of the dying, providing high quality care tailored to the patient's individual needs. We found a double challenge: to keep the original instrument as pure as possible, but to consider the context where it will be applied. Human resources; available drugs and routes of administration; Latin American cultural perspective on caring and dying; health care education; and translation barriers were some of the most important topics that we had to considered when we began the important task of implementing the LCP in this region of the world. A specific reality of our health system is that there are more specialist physicians than general practitioners, and even more doctors than nurses—an inverted pyramid. There is an enormous need to modify this ratio and redefine roles and tasks in order to develop a pathway focused on a multidisciplinary and multidimensional care.

The LCP is really becoming a new bridge between the port of Liverpool and that of Buenos Aires in South America, contributing to the increasing number of people who can get proper care and relief from end of life suffering.

Prof. Dr Gustavo de Simone, Medical Director of Pallium Latinoamerica (NGO).
Founder member of Arg Assoc of Pall Care

Dr Vilma Tripodoro, Coordinator of PC Section, Lanari Institute, Universidad de Buenos Aires. Past President of Arg Assoc of Pall Care

International perspective

LCP in Slovenia: experiences in implementing the LCP in Slovenia

In Slovenia, with a population of two million, approximately 18 000 deaths are registered per year. Palliative care is not yet well developed in Slovenia; there are only three palliative care units in three hospitals and a few palliative care teams in other health care settings; seven hospices, but only one with an inpatient unit. A National Plan for Palliative Care has been adapted in 2010, supported by an Action Plan for the next five years.

With the intention to support the development of palliative care in all settings and to foster an awareness of the need for education and teamwork, the introduction of the LCP was initiated with version 11 in 2007. It was successfully accepted in two teaching hospitals: the Oncology institute in Ljubljana and the University Clinic for Respiratory and Allergic Diseases, Golnik. There are numerous other settings in hospitals, community, and nursing homes where implementation has recently started.

In 2009 a pilot study introducing standard documentation and education into the institutions of all three levels of health care system in three regions was undertaken by the lead of a professional committee at the Ministry of Health; LCP was included in this standard documentation. Preliminary analysis shows encouraging results in terms of better symptom control, communication, satisfaction of patients' relatives and team members, and greater awareness of the need for continuous education.

Team members recognized the following most important advantages that supported the implementation:

- Criteria in place for the introduction of LCP made team members more confident in their work
- Forward planning and drug prescription in the community and in the nursing care setting was recognized as a very helpful procedure
- A clear decision point for withdrawing unnecessary drugs and procedures was recognized as very helpful
- Communication was supported by the LCP on appropriate timing

Family members recognized the following:

- Communication was much better than they had previously experienced from health care services

- ◆ When a patient started on the LCP, the meeting of a team member with the family was a turning point, helping them to understand the whole dying process

The main challenge was a very low awareness about palliative care among the majority of health care professionals and the public, which was recognized as a huge barrier to the implementation of the LCP. In summary:

- Lack of communication skills and authoritative relationships in the health care system made it difficult for the advantages of the LCP in terms of autonomy, and cooperation of patients and family members to be accepted
- Lack of effective team work among different health care professions meant the work mainly fell to the nurses
- Implementation takes time, additional manpower, and ongoing drive
- Documentation brings a new perspective of focus on the patient, which is the core driving force for change in attitudes

Dr Urska Lunder, Palliative Care Clinician, Director, Palliative Care Development Institute

Phase 2: Implementation

The local steering group will meet to discuss the LCP and customize prompts according to local need. It is important that the goals of care on the LCP remain unchanged to enable benchmarking in the future. Supportive documentation will need to be identified and leaflets produced. The LCP Central Team can support each organization to undertake a Base Review (retrospective audit) electronically (see Chapter 9).

An intensive induction education programme within at least the pilot site should be implemented so that 80% of the staff within the clinical area are aware of the LCP project plans before the LCP is implemented. The LCP Central Team advises that an LCP Resource Folder is available at local clinical level. Any existing learning and support mechanisms should be used at this time. A status report should be sent to the LCP Central Team and regular teleconference calls are very helpful.

International perspective

The LCP in India

The success of the Liverpool Care Pathway in the UK has led to considerations of its use internationally. In India, despite examples of high quality practice, less than 2% of the population can access the palliative care services they need. A project was initiated in 2006 to adapt the LCP and create a generic document for use in the Indian setting. The aims were:

- To improve existing services through the process of setting standards of best practice and audit
- To facilitate the spread of skills between palliative care services (specialist-specialist)
- To facilitate the sharing of skills and knowledge from specialist palliative care services and general health care settings (specialist-generalist)
- To develop the pathway as an education tool for use in both specialist and general settings

The pathway was redesigned and piloted in four sites in India and the results have been presented at national and international conferences. The national organization, the Indian Association of Palliative Care (IAPC) has formally endorsed the programme and the next phase of recruitment of new centres is currently underway.

Dr Libby Sallnow, Palliative Care Registrar, Barts and the London NHS Trust, UK
Dr Stanley Macaden, Retired CEO Bangalore Baptist Hospital, Bangalore, India

Phase 3: Dissemination

Each time the LCP is completed the lead clinician should review it and reflect on success and challenges within the local heath economy. Data from the first 20 LCPs once completed can be uploaded onto the electronic data capture tool with the support of LCP Central Team, and progress reviewed and disseminated. For some organizations where pilot work only has been undertaken a decision will need to be made by the steering group as to the next stage of dissemination. A wider dissemination and sustainability model will need to be considered and include the following areas for discussion, managerial and service improvement agenda, the learning and teaching plans for future ongoing programmes, and a future measurement and research agenda to maintain momentum and support organizational change. A clear decision and programme of work will need to be agreed if there is a decision to disseminate the LCP across the organization or institution beyond the pilot site(s).

International perspective

The LCP in Norway

Experiences with the translation:

When you feel that a valuable tool has been found, you really want to rush into using it. That is not possible, however, due to the required formal translation process. Looking back, we acknowledge the value of the translation period. This was the time to get to know the pathway, almost with a magnifying glass. Simultaneously we worked on the supporting documents and the implementation strategy. Our 'Just in case' safety box for home deaths was developed in this period and is widely used today. The whole process took us almost a year, but was really worth it.

Challenges:

The English and Norwegian languages have many similarities, but some of the core expressions do not have Norwegian counterparts. To give an example, there is no direct translation of the English word 'care', a longer expression must be used. The central words 'achieved' and 'variance' cannot be used in Norwegian in this context, so we have to use 'yes' and 'no' answers as to whether or not the goals are achieved. Answering the goals with negations has proved a practical challenge, as Norwegians usually express themselves the other way round!

First experience with implementation:

We had a flying start to our implementation. The management, both of the hospital and the medical department, as well as the staff on the busy wards were very interested to start using the LCP, especially after we had done the base reviews. One of the nurses approached us very eagerly in the hallway on the official starting day, telling that they had a candidate patient on the ward and had been preparing for the LCP during the weekend.

We find it crucial to have dedicated nurses and doctors available for support and help during the first months of implementation. As one of the younger nurses said, 'I find it challenging to work with dying patients, but you and the LCP help me get it right'.

The Regional Centre of Excellence for Palliative Care, Western Norway, has been responsible for coordinating the translation process and is also responsible for the further implementation.

Grethe Skorpen Iversen, RN (palliative care nurse), Regional Centre of Excellence for Palliative Care, Western Norway

International perspective

LCP in Italy: a strategy between dissemination and evaluation

The original LCP documentation for hospital and hospice (version 11) was translated into Italian and approved by the LCP Central Team UK, Marie Curie Palliative Care Institute Liverpool (MCPCIL) in 2007 and 2009 respectively. LCP was successfully piloted, and the process of implementation assessed with a mixed approach, in the general medicine ward of Villa Scassi Hospital in Genoa. At the time of writing, LCP has been registered and introduced in five hospital wards (four medical and one respiratory disease) and in 12 hospices from six Italian regions.

The Italian general strategy is a mixture of assessment and dissemination of the LCP programme. Assessment, in agreement with the framework for the evaluation of complex interventions proposed by the Medical Research Council includes both qualitative and quantitative approaches with different levels of complexity. The phase I study focusing on the process of implementation of the LCP Programme in seven Italian hospices has been completed, showing the feasibility of LCP implementation into the Italian context. A phase II study aimed at assessing the impact of introducing LCP in all Ligurian hospices was funded by Liguria Region (starting 2010).

Positive results from the pilot process of implementation in hospital and preliminary results from Italian and international phase I and II studies, encouraged us to design a cluster trial to evaluate the effectiveness of the LCP-I Programme in improving the quality of end of life care provided to cancer patients who die on hospital medical wards. The trial was registered and started in 2010 (ClinicalTrials.gov Identifier: NCT01081899). Final results should be available for 2012.

Three research projects funded by the Minister of Health and by Liguria Region with the aim of assessing the LCP are ongoing, and will allow better definition of the components of the LCP Programme. Specific materials for monitoring and evaluating the process of implementation were developed.

Massimo Costantini, MD, Head, Regional Palliative Care Network, National Cancer Research Institute, Genoa (Italy)

Many organizations or institutions will decide to continue a plan of dissemination across their organization with no future plans to work across sector or with other organizations at the current time.

International perspective

LCP German collaboration: Switzerland—Germany—Austria

Primarily, the LCP has been regarded as a tool for a fundamental change of culture, especially regarding inter-professional collaboration within hospitals and other care settings. In addition, this tool helps to demonstrate that palliative care has to offer more than empathy and listening, and requires a pragmatic approach and guidance for difficult clinical situations.

Both issues have been highlighted throughout the implementation of LCP in the German speaking countries. Nurses appreciate most the ability to demand inter-professional decision making and collaboration, and family members give positive feedback regarding improved quality of communication, information, and team consistency.

With all German speaking countries having a federal health care system with the lack of 'national guidance', the implementation of LCP within different care settings depends on an 'institution by institution' strategy. The German collaborative group therefore tries to keep all users tied collaboratively together in order to provide a chance for future benchmarking and international collaboration. It remains a challenge and an opportunity to translate the original document and approach into national 'culture' and professional behaviour and roles which are still very much hierarchical and dominated by 'medical' reasoning and leadership.

Steffen Eychmueller, MD, Head, Center for Palliative Care, Cantonal Hospital StGallen, Switzerland

Prof. Raymond Voltz, Department of Palliative Medicine, University Hospital Cologne, Germany

---

Phase 4: Sustainability

This phase will support the steering group to embed the LCP Continuous Quality Improvement Programme across the organization or institution. A clear decision and associated plan will need to be agreed with the LCP Central Team if the organization or institution is planning for a wider dissemination programme within a research based framework beyond the organization or institution, but led by the key stakeholders or steering group from within the organization. There will be a clear quality initiative to recognize this LCP programme within the mainstream health care agenda across the local health economy in all care settings.

There are many examples of countries who have implemented and disseminated the LCP programme across the health economy with best practice examples across care settings but without a future intention to develop an approach to become a national LCP office.

International perspective

The LCP in Sweden

The LCP implementation in Sweden is coordinated from the research and development unit at Stiftelsen Stockholms Sjukhem in Stockholm. At the end of 2009, 80 units were registered as using LCP at different stages of implementation. Among these were palliative care inpatient units and hospices, palliative home care teams, hospital wards, and community care and nursing homes. Almost all patient documentation in Sweden is electronic using many different systems. It is a great challenge to have LCP integrated into these different systems, few of which have been designed to support a pathway- or process-oriented way of documentation.

Professor Carl Johan Fürst MD PhD, Professor/Medical Director, Stockholms Sjukhem
   Foundation, Sweden

International perspective

The LCP in the Netherlands

After the translation of the LCP into Dutch the effect of the LCP was studied in relation to the quality of life in the last three days of life; to the communication and the bereavement process; and to the quality of documentation in the last three days of life. Almost 500 patients were included in this study which showed that the LCP contributes to decline in symptom burden for dying patients; to lower levels of bereavement in the relatives; and to better quality documentation. Based on these results the implementation of the LCP across all care settings was enhanced and coordinated by the Comprehensive Cancer Centre Rotterdam. Twice a year a foundation course is given which is supported by training on the job. A meeting of all institutions working with the LCP is organized every year to share experiences and to discuss the content of care. The national implementation programme was launched in collaboration with the other seven comprehensive cancer centres and was financially supported by the Ministry of Health, Welfare, and Sports. National products were developed consisting of the three versions of the LCP (Home care, Nursing home, and Hospital); education programmes; and a website: *www.zorgpadstervensfase.nl.* A national reference group is supporting the national implementation programme. Fifty organizations have been working with the LCP for some time and at least a further fifty organizations are in the middle of the implementation process.

The whole process from translation to national implementation was an impressive and motivating experience. A lot of caregivers can't wait to implement and work with the LCP. The big challenge we are now facing is to develop the national implementation programme without losing the essence of the LCP: continuous improvement of care for the dying patient in all care settings.

Dr Lia Van Zuylen (MD,PhD), Medical Oncologist/Coordinator of Palliative Care Team, Erasmus MC University Hospital, Rotterdam, the Netherlands

Development of a State/Country/National LCP Office

At this stage there will need to be a full project plan in place agreed by key stakeholders and fully endorsed by the LCP Central Team. There will need to be national recognition of a key institution or organization leading on this agenda; this will include a national resource written into a contractual agreement with academic support in view of the ongoing learning, teaching, research, and innovation portfolio.

A national lead clinician will be required and depending on the size of the country or population served more than one office may be required. The ongoing design of the LCP and all associated materials including a national core LCP document that is fully compliant with the current core document held by the LCP Central Team will be driven by this national office with the ongoing support of the LCP Central Team. Each national office will have a licence and contract from the LCP Central Team but this may differ across countries and the needs of each will always be individualized.

Conclusion

It has been demonstrated that the LCP is transferable for use in other languages and within very different cultural contexts. Since 2004 an annual LCP international meeting has attracted attendance across 20 countries. Doctors,

The international perspective

The LCP in New Zealand (NZ)

In collaboration with the LCP Central Team, New Zealand (NZ) established the first national LCP office outside of the UK to promote and coordinate sustainable implementation of the LCP. The NZ LCP Office is funded by the NZ Ministry of Health and is underpinned by NZ's palliative care strategy (7) that recommends equitable access to quality end of life care for all dying people in NZ. A major achievement of the NZ LCP office has been an evaluation of its role and ongoing value, based on key stakeholder perspectives. Key LCP stakeholders reported that access to staff knowledgeable about the context of the LCP and end of life care in NZ was highly valued. Participants appreciated the NZ LCP Office working alongside LCP facilitators at all stages of the LCP journey bridging the gap between the theory and actual implementation of the LCP, and in developing a national LCP information network. The evaluation also revealed that the participants felt that the NZ LCP Office could provide political influence and a strategic voice for end of life care policy and service development. A major challenge for us was identifying and addressing ad hoc implementation plans and the use of non-compliant LCP documents that preceded the development of the NZ LCP Office; which risked diluting and compromising the effectiveness and sustainability of the LCP over time. Within the first year of operation, the Ministry of Health agreed to provide the NZ LCP Office with ongoing funding and commended the office for providing a fantastic service that had already made significant improvements in the quality and consistency of care of the dying in NZ.

Theresa MacKenzie, National Liverpool Care Pathway (LCP) Lead–NZ, Arohanui
    Hospice, Palmerston North, New Zealand

nurses, social workers, psychologists, researchers, and other professionals come together to share experiences of the LCP programme and the LCP model itself. Communities, sometimes small, growing slowly into local and regional groups gathering once a year, have started to learn together to share experiences. It has been interesting to explore together intrinsic habits, childhood learning, traditions, cultures, and shared and non shared beliefs. The context of patient and family is core for some cultures yet alien to others. In most western countries the patient wherever possible has the right to dictate what is shared with his family or not; however, in other cultures it is the family who dictates what a patient should or should not know. Pain maybe something to be controlled to promote comfort or on the other hand must be experienced to promote spiritual wellbeing.

The best quality of care in the last hours or days of life is a basic human right that transcends cultural beliefs and boundaries. The LCP serves to encompass the four key domains of care ie physical, psychological, social, and spiritual which are intrinsic in care of the dying. Individual patient preferences and belief systems can then be reflected and documented accordingly. The LCP can support the cultural norms that exist within an individual country.

Although each participating individual or country at the international meeting is divided by implementation phases, all speak a similar international language, though for most of the group, English is not their mother tongue, yet, a common frame of reference is emerging. The communication is about something else that starts to resonate beyond the sometimes awkward words. Sharing and learning from each other allows for helping to learn as fast as possible, because we share the notion that a dignified death is the last good thing we can do for a person, before s/he has to leave us. And as we are all from a different age, I am sure that some of us also hope that if we are capable of helping to make care for the dying better now, we ourselves, one day, hope to benefit from that.

References

1 Ferris FD, Balfour HM, Bowen K, et al. A model to guide patient and family care: based on nationally accepted principles and norms of practice. *J PainSymptom Manage* 2002;**24**:106–23.

2 National Consensus Project for Quality Palliative Care. *Clinical Practice Guidelines for Quality Palliative Care*, 2009 Second Edition. http://www.nationalconsensusproject.org (accessed 6 July 2010).

3 Davies E, Higginson IJ eds.(2004). *Better palliative care for older people*. World Health Organization Europe, http://www.euro.who.int/document/E82933.pdf (Accessed 20 March 2010)

4 Council of Europe (2003). *Recommendation 24 of the Committee of Ministers to member states on the organization of palliative care*,http://www.coe.int/t/dg3/health/Source/Rec(2003)24_en.pdf (accessed 7 April 2010).

5 Cull A, Sprangers M, Bjordal K, Aaronson N, *on behalf of the EORTC Quality of Life Study Group EORTC Quality of Life Study Group Translation Procedure* July 1998 EORTC, Brussels.

6 Edwards-Deming W. (1994) *The new economics for industry, government, education.* 2nd ed. Massachusetts Institute of Technology Centre for Advanced Engineering Study Massachusetts.

7 Minister of Health (2001). *New Zealand Palliative Care Strategy*. Ministry of Health: Wellington.

Appendix 1

Liverpool Care Pathway for the Dying Patient (LCP)
supporting care in the last hours or days of life

Introduction

The aim of the LCP continuous quality improvement programme is to translate the excellent model of hospice care for the dying into other health care settings using an integrated care pathway (ICP) for the last hours or days of life.

The implementation of the programme will create a change in the organisation. Recognition of the fundamental aspects of a change management programme is pivotal to success. The Service Improvement Model used at the Marie Curie Palliative Care Institute Liverpool (MCPCIL) is a 4-phased approach incorporating a 10-step continuous quality improvement process for the LCP Programme that can be downloaded from the web site www.mcpcil.org.uk

The LCP generic document is only as good as the teams using it. Using the LCP generic document in any environment therefore requires regular assessment and involves regular reflection, challenge, critical senior decision-making and clinical skill, in the best interest of the patient. A robust continuous learning and teaching programme must underpin the implementation and dissemination of the LCP generic document. The LCP generic version 11 has been reviewed since December 2007 as part of an extensive consultation exercise and LCP generic version 12 is now available to reflect the feedback from the consultation and latest evidence.

The ethos of the LCP generic version 12 document has remained unchanged. In response to the consultation exercise including 2 rounds of the National Care of the Dying Audit – Hospitals (NCDAH), version 12 has greater clarity in key areas particularly communication, nutrition and hydration. Care of the dying patient and their relative or carer can be supported effectively by either version of the LCP. The responsibility for the use of the LCP generic document as part of a continuous quality improvement programme sits within the governance of an organisation underpinned by a robust ongoing education and training programme.

We believe as with any evolving tool or technology that those organisations who are using the LCP generic version 11 will work towards adopting version 12.

LCP CORE DOCUMENTATION	
LCP generic document version 12:	**Supporting information:**
o Relative or carer information	o Relative or carer information leaflet
o Algorithm regarding decision making	o Healthcare professional information
o Initial assessment	o Medication guidance
o Ongoing assessment	o Facilities leaflet
o Care after death	o Coping with dying leaflet
o Variance analysis	o Grieving leaflet
	o Helpful reference list

As with all clinical guidelines and pathways the LCP aims to support but does not
replace clinical judgement.

Liverpool Care Pathway for the Dying Patient (LCP)
supporting care in the last hours or days of life

Information sheet to be given to the relative or carer following a discussion regarding the plan of care.

The doctors and nurses will have explained to you that there has been a change in your relative or friend's condition. They believe that the person you care about is now dying and in the last hours or days of life.

The LCP is a document which supports the doctors and nurses to give the best quality of care. All care will be reviewed regularly.

You and your relative or friend will be involved in the discussion regarding the plan of care with the aim that you fully understand the reasons why decisions are being made. If your relative or friend's condition improves then the plan of care will be reviewed and changed. All decisions will be reviewed regularly. If after a discussion with the doctors and nurses you do not agree with any decisions you may want to ask for a second opinion.

Communication

There are information leaflets available for you as it is sometimes difficult to remember everything at this sad and challenging time. The doctors and nurses will ask you for your contact details, as keeping you updated is a priority.

Medication

Medicine that is not helpful at this time may be stopped and new medicines prescribed. Medicines for symptom control will only be given when needed, at the right time and just enough and no more than is needed to help the symptom.

Comfort

The doctors and nurses will not want to interrupt your time with your relative or friend. They will make sure that as far as possible any needs at this time are met. Please let them know if you feel those needs are not being met, for whatever reason.

You can support care in important ways such as spending time together, sharing memories and news of family and friends.

LCP generic version 12 – December 2009   ADD NAME OF ORGANISATION HERE
© Marie Curie Palliative Care Institute Liverpool (MCPCIL)

Information sheet to be given to the relative or carer continued:

Reduced need for food and drink

Loss of interest in and a reduced need for food and drink is part of the normal dying process. When a person stops eating & drinking it can be hard to accept even when we know they are dying. Your relative or friend will be supported to eat and drink for as long as possible. If they cannot take fluids by mouth, fluids given by a drip may be considered.

Fluids given by a drip will only be used where it is helpful and not harmful. This decision will be explained to your relative or friend if possible and to you.

Good mouth care is very important at this time. The nurses will explain to you how mouth care is given and may ask if you would like to help them give this care.

> **Caring well for your relative or friend is important to us. Please speak to the doctors or nurses if there are any questions that occur to you, no matter how insignificant you think they may be or how busy the staff may seem. This may all be very unfamiliar to you and we are here to explain, support and care.**

We can be reached during daytimes at:..

Night time at:...

Other information or contact numbers (e.g. palliative care nurse / district nurse):
....
....
....
....
....

This space can be used for you to list any questions you may want to ask the doctors and nurses:
....
....
....
....
....

LCP generic version 12 – December 2009
© Marie Curie Palliative Care Institute Liverpool (MCPCIL)

ADD NAME OF ORGANISATION HERE

Name:.. NHS no:.. Date:...............................

Liverpool Care Pathway for the Dying Patient (LCP)
supporting care in the last hours or days of life

Location: (e.g. hospital, ward, care home etc.):...

As with all clinical guidelines and pathways the LCP aims to support but does not replace clinical judgement

- ❑ The LCP generic document guides and enables healthcare professionals to focus on care in the last hours or days of life. This provides high quality care tailored to the patient's individual needs, when their death is expected.

- ❑ Using the LCP in any environment requires regular assessment and involves regular reflection, challenge, critical senior decision-making and clinical skill, in the best interest of the patient. A robust continuous learning and teaching programme must underpin the use of the LCP.

- ❑ The recognition and diagnosis of dying is always complex; irrespective of previous diagnosis or history. Uncertainty is an integral part of dying. There are occasions when a patient who is thought to be dying lives longer than expected and vice versa. Seek a second opinion or specialist palliative care support as needed.

- ❑ Changes in care at this complex, uncertain time are made in the best interest of the patient and relative or carer and needs to be reviewed regularly by the multidisciplinary team (MDT).

- ❑ Good comprehensive clear communication is pivotal and all decisions leading to a change in care delivery should be communicated to the patient where appropriate and to the relative or carer. The views of all concerned must be listened to and documented.

- ❑ If a goal on the LCP is not achieved this should be coded as a variance. This is not a negative process but demonstrates the individual nature of the patient's condition based on their particular needs, your clinical judgement and the needs of the relative or carer.

- ❑ The LCP does not preclude the use of clinically assisted nutrition or hydration or antibiotics. All clinical decisions must be made in the patient's best interest.

- ❑ A blanket policy of clinically assisted (artificial) nutrition or hydration, or of no clinically assisted (artificial) hydration, is ethically indefensible and in the case of patients lacking capacity prohibited under the Mental Capacity Act (2005).

- ❑ For the purpose of this LCP generic version 12 document - The term best interest includes medical, physical, emotional, social and spiritual and all other factors relevant to the patient's welfare.

The patient will be assessed regularly and a formal full MDT review must be undertaken every 3 days.

The responsibility for the use of the LCP generic document as part of a continuous quality improvement programme sits within the governance of an organisation and must be underpinned by a robust education and training programme.

References:
Ellershaw and Wilkinson Eds (2003) *Care of the dying: A pathway to excellence.* Oxford: Oxford University Press.
National Institute for Clinical Excellence (2004) Improving Supportive and Palliative Care for Adults with Cancer. London, NICE
MCPCIL (2009) National Care of the Dying Audit Hospitals Generic Report Round 2. www.mcpcil.org.uk

LCP generic version 12 – December 2009   ADD NAME OF ORGANISATION HERE
© Marie Curie Palliative Care Institute Liverpool (MCPCIL)

Name:.. NHS no:... Date:..

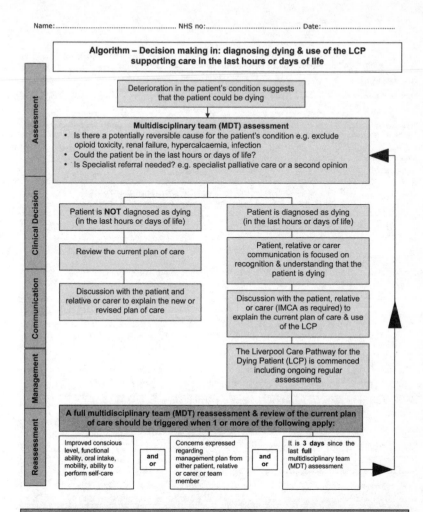

Algorithm – Decision making in: diagnosing dying & use of the LCP supporting care in the last hours or days of life

Assessment

Deterioration in the patient's condition suggests that the patient could be dying

Multidisciplinary team (MDT) assessment
- Is there a potentially reversible cause for the patient's condition e.g. exclude opioid toxicity, renal failure, hypercalcaemia, infection
- Could the patient be in the last hours or days of life?
- Is Specialist referral needed? e.g. specialist palliative care or a second opinion

Clinical Decision

Patient is **NOT** diagnosed as dying (in the last hours or days of life)

Patient is diagnosed as dying (in the last hours or days of life)

Review the current plan of care

Patient, relative or carer communication is focused on recognition & understanding that the patient is dying

Communication

Discussion with the patient and relative or carer to explain the new or revised plan of care

Discussion with the patient, relative or carer (IMCA as required) to explain the current plan of care & use of the LCP

Management

The Liverpool Care Pathway for the Dying Patient (LCP) is commenced including ongoing regular assessments

Reassessment

A full multidisciplinary team (MDT) reassessment & review of the current plan of care should be triggered when 1 or more of the following apply:

| Improved conscious level, functional ability, oral intake, mobility, ability to perform self-care | **and or** | Concerns expressed regarding management plan from either patient, relative or carer or team member | **and or** | It is **3 days** since the last **full** multidisciplinary team (MDT) assessment |

Always remember that the Specialist Palliative Care Team are there for advice and support, especially if: Symptom control is difficult and/or if there are difficult communication issues or you need advice or support regarding your care delivery supported by the LCP

LCP generic version 12 – December 2009
© Marie Curie Palliative Care Institute Liverpool (MCPCIL)   ADD NAME OF ORGANISATION HERE

Name:... NHS no:.. Date:.................................

Healthcare professional documenting the MDT decision

Following a full MDT assessment and a decision to use the LCP:

Date LCP commenced:..

Time LCP commenced:..

Name (Print):..................................... Signature:...................................

This will vary according to circumstances and local governance arrangements. In general this should be the most senior healthcare professional immediately available.

The decision must be endorsed by the most senior healthcare professional responsible for the patient's care at the earliest opportunity if different from above.

Name (Print):..................................... Signature:...................................

All personnel completing the LCP please sign below
You should also have read and understood the guidance on pages 1 - 2

Name (print)	Full signature	Initials	Professional title	Date

Record all full MDT reassessments here (including full formal MDT reassessment every 3 days)

Reassessment date:....................................... Reassessment time:...

Reassessment date:....................................... Reassessment time:...

Reassessment date:....................................... Reassessment time:...

Reassessment date:....................................... Reassessment time:...

If the LCP is discontinued please record here:

Date LCP discontinued.. Time LCP discontinued...

Reasons why the LCP was discontinued:...

....

....

Decision to discontinue the LCP shared with the patient   Yes ☐   No ☐

Decision to discontinue the LCP shared with the relative or carer   Yes ☐   No ☐

Name:.. NHS no:... Date:...

Section 1   Initial assessment (joint assessment by doctor and nurse)

Diagnosis & Baseline Information

DIAGNOSIS:.. Co-morbidity:...
.... Ethnicity:......................................
DOB:..............................   Age:...........   NHS no:....................................   Female ☐ Male ☐

At the time of the assessment is the patient:

In pain	Yes ☐ No ☐	Able to swallow	Yes ☐ No ☐	Confused	Yes ☐ No ☐
Agitated	Yes ☐ No ☐	Continent (bladder)	Yes ☐ No ☐	*(record below which is applicable)*	
Nauseated	Yes ☐ No ☐	Catheterised	Yes ☐ No ☐	Conscious	☐
Vomiting	Yes ☐ No ☐	Continent (bowels)	Yes ☐ No ☐	Semi-conscious	☐
Dyspnoeic	Yes ☐ No ☐	Constipated	Yes ☐ No ☐	Unconscious	☐
Experiencing respiratory tract secretions			Yes ☐ No ☐		
Experiencing other symptoms (e.g. oedema, itch)			Yes ☐ No ☐		

Communication

Goal 1.1: The patient is able to take a full and active part in communication

         Achieved ☐   Variance ☐   Unconscious ☐

Barriers that have the potential to prevent communication have been assessed

First language...   Other issues identified..

Consider need for an interpreter: (contact no) ....

Other barriers to communication...

Consider: Hearing, vision, speech, learning disabilities, dementia (use of assessment tools), neurological conditions and confusion

The relative or carer may know how specific signs indicate distress if the patient is unable to articulate their own concerns

Does the patient have:-

An advance care plan?

An expressed wish for organ/tissue donation?

An advance decision to refuse treatment (ADRT)?

Does the patient have the capacity to make their own decisions on their own treatment at this moment in time?

consider the support of an IMCA – if required document below:

Comments:..
....

Goal 1.2: The relative or carer is able to take a full and active part in communication   Achieved ☐   Variance ☐

First language...   Other Issues identified..

Consider need for an interpreter (contact no):...

Other barriers to communication:...

Goal 1.3: The patient is aware that they are dying   Achieved ☐   Variance ☐   Unconscious ☐

Goal 1.4: The relative or carer is aware that the patient is dying   Achieved ☐   Variance ☐

Goal 1.5: The Clinical team have up to date contact information for the relative or carer as documented below

         Achieved ☐   Variance ☐

1st contact name:...

Relationship to the patient:...   Tel no:.............................   Mobile no:...........................

When to contact: At any time ☐   Not at night-time ☐   Staying with the patient overnight ☐

2nd contact:..

Relationship to the patient:...   Tel no:.............................   Mobile no:...........................

When to contact: At any time ☐   Not at night-time ☐   Staying with patient the overnight ☐

Next of kin - this may be different from above   N/A ☐   **Lasting Power of Attorney (LPA) (if applicable)**   N/A ☐

Name:...   Name:...

Contact details:...   Contact details:...

....

....

Name:.. NHS no:.. Date:.............................

Section 1	Initial assessment (joint assessment by doctor and nurse)

Facilities

Goal 2: The relative or carer has had a full explanation of the facilities available to them and a facilities leaflet has been given   Achieved ☐   Variance ☐

Facilities may include: car parking, toilet, bathroom facilities, beverages, payphone, accommodation

Eg. Community Setting - In the patient's own home this could include access details to the district nursing team, palliative care team , out of hours services, GP, home loans, what to do in an emergency, oxygen supplies

Spirituality

Goal 3.1: The patient is given the opportunity to discuss what is important to them at this time eg. their wishes, feelings, faith , beliefs, values   Achieved ☐   Variance ☐   Unconscious ☐

Patient may be anxious for self or others. Consider specific religious and cultural needs

Consider music, art, poetry, reading, photographs, something that has been important to the belief system or the well-being of the patient

Did the patient take the opportunity to discuss the above   Yes ☐   No ☐   Unconscious ☐

Religious tradition identified, please specify: ....

Support of the chaplaincy team offered   Yes ☐   No ☐

If no give reason:...

In-house support   Tel/bleep no: ....Name: ....   Date/time: ....

External support   Tel/bleep no: ....Name: ....   Date/time: ....

Needs now:...

....

....

....

Needs at death:...

....

Needs after death:...

....

....

Goal 3.2: The relative or carer is given the opportunity to discuss what is important to them at this time e.g. their wishes, feelings, faith, beliefs, values   Achieved ☐   Variance ☐

Comments..

....

....

Did the relative or carer take the opportunity to discuss the above   Yes ☐   No ☐

Medication

Goal 4.1: The patient has medication prescribed on a prn basis for all of the following 5 symptoms which may develop in the last hours or days of life   Achieved ☐   Variance ☐

Pain   ☐

Agitation   ☐

Respiratory tract secretions   ☐

Nausea / Vomiting   ☐

Dyspnoea   ☐

Anticipatory prescribing in this manner will ensure that there is no delay in responding to a symptom if it occurs

Current Medication assessed and non essentials discontinued

Medicines for symptom control will only be given when needed, at the right time and just enough and no more than is needed to help the symptom

Goal 4.2: Equipment is available for the patient to support a continuous subcutaneous infusion (CSCI) of medication where required

     Achieved ☐   Variance ☐   Already in place ☐   Not required ☐

If a CSCI is to be used explain the rationale to the patient, relative or carer. Not all patients who are dying will require a CSCI

Name:.. NHS no:.. Date:..

Section 1   Initial assessment (joint assessment by doctor and nurse)

Current Interventions

Goal 5.1: The patient's need for current interventions has been reviewed by the MDT   Achieved ☐ Variance ☐

	Currently not being taken/ or given	Discontinued	Continued	Commenced
5a: Routine blood tests	☐	☐	☐	
5b: Intravenous antibiotics	☐	☐	☐	☐
5c: Blood glucose monitoring	☐	☐	☐	
5d: Recording of routine vital signs	☐	☐	☐	
5e: Oxygen therapy	☐	☐	☐	☐

5.2: The patient has a Do Not Attempt Cardiopulmonary Resuscitation Order in place   Achieved ☐ Variance ☐
Please complete the appropriate associated documentation according to policy and procedure
Explain to the patient, relative or carer as appropriate

5.3: Implantable Cardioverter Defibrillator (ICD) is deactivated   Achieved ☐ Variance ☐ No ICD in place ☐
Contact the patient's cardiologist. Refer to the ECG technician & refer to local/ regional - policy/procedure.
Information leaflet given to the patient, relative or carer as appropriate

Nutrition

Goal 6: The need for clinically assisted (artificial) nutrition is reviewed by the MDT   Achieved ☐ Variance ☐
The patient should be supported to take food by mouth for as long as tolerated
For many patients the use of clinically assisted (artificial) nutrition will not be required
A reduced need for food is part of the normal dying process
If clinically assisted (artificial) nutrition is already in place please record route   NG ☐ PEG/PEJ ☐ NJ ☐ TPN ☐
Is clinically assisted (artificial) nutrition   Not required ☐ Discontinued ☐ Continued ☐
Consider reduction in rate / volume according to individual need if nutritional support is in place
Explain the plan of care to the patient where appropriate, and to the relative or carer

Hydration

Goal 7: The need for clinically assisted (artificial) hydration is reviewed by the MDT   Achieved ☐ Variance ☐
The patient should be supported to take fluids by mouth for as long as tolerated
For many patients the use of clinically assisted (artificial) hydration will not be required
A reduced need for fluids is part of the normal dying process
Symptoms of thirst / dry mouth do not always indicate dehydration but are often due to mouth breathing or medication. Good mouth care is essential
If clinically assisted (artificial) hydration is already in place please record route   IV ☐ S/C ☐ PEG/PEJ ☐ NG ☐
Is clinically assisted (artificial) hydration   Not required ☐ Discontinued ☐ Continued ☐ Commenced ☐
Consider reduction in rate / volume according to individual need if hydration support is in place. If required consider the s/c route
Explain the plan of care to the patient where appropriate, and the relative or carer

Skin Care

Goal 8: The patient's skin integrity is assessed   Achieved ☐ Variance ☐
The aim is to prevent pressure ulcers or further deterioration if a pressure ulcer is present. Use a recognised risk assessment tool
e.g. Waterlow / Braden to support clinical judgement. The frequency of repositioning should be determined by skin inspection,
assessment and the patient's individual needs. Consider the use of special aids (mattress / bed)
Record the plan of care on the initial assessment MDT sheet where appropriate

Explanation of the plan of care

Goal 9.1: A full explanation of the current plan of care (LCP) is given to the patient
   Achieved ☐ Variance ☐ Unconscious ☐

Goal 9.2: A full explanation of the current plan of care (LCP) is given to the relative or carer
   Achieved ☐ Variance ☐
Name of relative or carer(s) present and relationship to the patient:...
....
Names of healthcare professionals present:...
Information sheet at front of the LCP or equivalent relative or carer information leaflet given   Yes ☐ No ☐
Parents or carer should be given or have access to age appropriate advice and information to support children/adolescents

Goal 9.3: The LCP Coping with dying leaflet or equivalent is given to the relative or carer
   Achieved ☐ Variance ☐

Goal 9.4: The patient's primary health care team / GP practice is notified that the patient is dying
   Achieved ☐ Variance ☐
G.P practice to be contacted if unaware that the patient is dying, message can be left or sent via a secure fax

If you have recorded a variance against any of the goals of care please record on the variance sheet, see page 8

Name:... NHS no:.. Date:......................................

Section 1	Initial assessment

<table>
<tr><td rowspan="4">Signatures</td><td colspan="2">Please sign here on completion of the initial assessment</td></tr>
<tr><td>Doctor's name (print):...........................</td><td>Nurse's name (print):.............................</td></tr>
<tr><td>Doctor's signature:................................</td><td>Nurse's signature:.................................</td></tr>
<tr><td>Date.................Time..............................</td><td>Date......................... Time.......................</td></tr>
</table>

Section 1 Initial assessment MDT progress notes

Date	Supportive information: Plan of care to monitor skin integrity, nutrition / hydration - include here any specific information regarding this patient; relative or carer that has not been captured in the initial assessment that you believe needs to be highlighted.

Name:.. NHS no:... Date:.............................

Variance analysis sheet for initial assessment

What variance occurred & why? (what was the issue?)	Action taken (what did you do?)	Outcome (did this solve the issue?)
Goal: Signature:.......................... Date / Time:.......................	Signature:.......................... Date / Time:.......................	Signature:.......................... Date / Time:.......................
Goal: Signature:.......................... Date / Time:.......................	Signature:.......................... Date / Time:.......................	Signature:.......................... Date / Time:.......................
Goal: Signature:.......................... Date / Time:.......................	Signature:.......................... Date / Time:.......................	Signature:.......................... Date / Time:.......................
Goal: Signature:.......................... Date / Time:.......................	Signature:.......................... Date / Time:.......................	Signature:.......................... Date / Time:.......................
Goal: Signature:.......................... Date / Time:.......................	Signature:.......................... Date / Time:.......................	Signature:.......................... Date / Time:.......................

Name:.. NHS no:... Date:....................................

Section 2   Ongoing assessment of the plan of care – LCP DAY........

Undertake an MDT assessment & review of the current management plan if:

Improved conscious level, functional ability, oral intake, mobility, ability to perform self-care	and or	Concern expressed regarding management plan from either the patient, relative or team member	and or	It is 3 days since the last full MDT assessment

Consider the support of the specialist palliative care team and/or a second opinion as required. Document all reassessment dates and times on page 3

Codes to be recorded at each timed assessment (a moment in time)   A= Achieved   V = Variance (exception reporting)

Record an A or a V not a signature	0400	0800	1200	1600	2000	2400
Goal a: The patient does not have pain Verbalised by patient if conscious, pain free on movement. Observe for non-verbal cues. Consider need for positional change. Use a pain assessment tool if appropriate. Consider prn analgesia for incident pain						
Goal b: The patient is not agitated Patient does not display signs of restlessness or distress, exclude reversible causes e.g. retention of urine, opioid toxicity						
Goal c: The patient does not have respiratory tract secretions Consider positional change. Discuss symptoms & plan of care with patient, relative or carer Medication to be given as soon as symptom occurs						
Goal d: The patient does not have nausea Verbalised by patient if conscious						
Goal e: The patient is not vomiting						
Goal f: The patient is not breathless Verbalised by patient if conscious, consider positional change. Use of a fan may be helpful						
Goal g: The patient does not have urinary problems Use of pads, urinary catheter as required						
Goal h: The patient does not have bowel problems Monitor – constipation / diarrhoea. Monitor skin integrity Bowels last opened:.........................						
Goal i: The patient does not have other symptoms Record symptom here... *If no other symptoms present please record N/A*						
Goal j: The patient's comfort & safety regarding the administration of medication is maintained If CSCI in place – monitoring sheet in progress S/C butterfly in place if needed for prn medication location:............................ The patient is only receiving medication that is beneficial at this time. *If no medication required please record N/A*						

LCP generic version 12 – December 2009
© Marie Curie Palliative Care Institute Liverpool (MCPCIL)

ADD NAME OF ORGANISATION HERE

Name:.. NHS no:.. Date:.......................................

Section 2   Ongoing assessment of the plan of care – LCP continued DAY....

Codes to be recorded at each timed assessment (a moment in time) A= Achieved   V = Variance (exception reporting)

	0400	0800	1200	1600	2000	2400
Goal k: The patient receives fluids to support their individual needs The patient is supported to take oral fluids / thickened fluids for as long as tolerated. Monitor for signs of aspiration and/or distress. If symptomatically dehydrated & not deemed futile, consider clinically assisted (artificial) hydration if in the patient's best interest. If in place monitor & review rate/volume. Explain the plan of care with the patient and relative or carer						
Goal l: The patient's mouth is moist and clean See mouth care policy. Relative or carer involved in care giving as appropriate. Mouth care tray at the bedside						
Goal m: The patient's skin integrity is maintained Assessment, cleansing, positioning, use of special aids (mattress / bed). The frequency of repositioning should be determined by skin inspection and the patient's individual needs. *Waterlow / Braden score:*....................						
Goal n: The patient's personal hygiene needs are met Skin care, wash, eye care, change of clothing according to individual needs. Relative or carer involved in care giving as appropriate						
Goal o: The patient receives their care in a physical environment adjusted to support their individual needs Well fitting curtains, screens, clean environment, sufficient space at bedside, consider fragrance, silence, music, light, dark, pictures, photographs, nurse call bell accessible						
Goal p: The patient's psychological well-being is maintained Staff just being at the bedside can be a sign of support and caring. Respectful verbal and non-verbal communication, use of listening skills, information and explanation of care given. Use of touch if appropriate. Spiritual/religious/cultural needs – consider support of the chaplaincy team						
Goal q: The well-being of the relative or carer attending the patient is maintained Just being at the bedside can be a sign of support and caring. Consider spiritual/religious/cultural needs, expressions may be unfamiliar to the healthcare professional but normal for the relative or carer – support of chaplaincy team may be helpful. Listen & respond to worries/fears. Age appropriate advice & information to support children/adolescents available to parents or carers. Allow the opportunity to reminisce. Offer a drink						
Signature of the person making the assessment						
Signature of the registered nurse per shift	Night	Early		Late		Night

LCP generic version 12 – December 2009
© Marie Curie Palliative Care Institute Liverpool (MCPCIL)

ADD NAME OF ORGANISATION HERE

Name:.. NHS no:.. Date:..

Section 2   Ongoing assessment of the plan of care – LCP DAY........

Undertake an MDT assessment & review of the current management plan if:

Improved conscious level, functional ability, oral intake, mobility, ability to perform self-care	and or	Concern expressed regarding management plan from either the patient, relative or team member	and or	It is 3 days since the last **full** MDT assessment

Consider the support of the specialist palliative care team and/or a second opinion as required. Document all reassessment dates and times on page 3

Codes to be recorded at each timed assessment (a moment in time)   A= Achieved   V = Variance (exception reporting)

Record an A or a V not a signature	0400	0800	1200	1600	2000	2400
Goal a: The patient does not have pain Verbalised by patient if conscious, pain free on movement. Observe for non-verbal cues. Consider need for positional change. Use a pain assessment tool if appropriate. Consider prn analgesia for incident pain						
Goal b: The patient is not agitated Patient does not display signs of restlessness or distress, exclude reversible causes e.g. retention of urine, opioid toxicity						
Goal c: The patient does not have respiratory tract secretions Consider positional change. Discuss symptoms & plan of care with patient, relative or carer Medication to be given as soon as symptom occurs						
Goal d: The patient does not have nausea Verbalised by patient if conscious						
Goal e: The patient is not vomiting						
Goal f: The patient is not breathless Verbalised by patient if conscious, consider positional change. Use of a fan may be helpful						
Goal g: The patient does not have urinary problems Use of pads, urinary catheter as required						
Goal h: The patient does not have bowel problems Monitor – constipation / diarrhoea. Monitor skin integrity Bowels last opened:.........................						
Goal i: The patient does not have other symptoms Record symptom here.. *If no other symptoms present please record N/A*						
Goal j: The patient's comfort & safety regarding the administration of medication is maintained If CSCI in place – monitoring sheet in progress S/C butterfly in place if needed for prn medication location:............................. The patient is only receiving medication that is beneficial at this time. *If no medication required please record N/A*						

Name:.. NHS no:.. Date:......................................

Section 2   Ongoing assessment of the plan of care – LCP continued DAY....

Codes to be recorded at each timed assessment (a moment in time) A= Achieved   V = Variance (exception reporting)

	0400	0800	1200	1600	2000	2400
Goal k: The patient receives fluids to support their individual needs The patient is supported to take oral fluids / thickened fluids for as long as tolerated. Monitor for signs of aspiration and/or distress. If symptomatically dehydrated & not deemed futile, consider clinically assisted (artificial) hydration if in the patient's best interest. If in place monitor & review rate/volume. Explain the plan of care with the patient and relative or carer						
Goal l: The patient's mouth is moist and clean See mouth care policy. Relative or carer involved in care giving as appropriate. Mouth care tray at the bedside						
Goal m: The patient's skin integrity is maintained Assessment, cleansing, positioning, use of special aids (mattress / bed). The frequency of repositioning should be determined by skin inspection and the patient's individual needs. *Waterlow / Braden score:*...................						
Goal n: The patient's personal hygiene needs are met Skin care, wash, eye care, change of clothing according to individual needs. Relative or carer involved in care giving as appropriate						
Goal o: The patient receives their care in a physical environment adjusted to support their individual needs Well fitting curtains, screens, clean environment, sufficient space at bedside, consider fragrance, silence, music, light, dark, pictures, photographs, nurse call bell accessible						
Goal p: The patient's psychological well-being is maintained Staff just being at the bedside can be a sign of support and caring. Respectful verbal and non-verbal communication, use of listening skills, information and explanation of care given. Use of touch if appropriate. Spiritual/religious/cultural needs – consider support of the chaplaincy team						
Goal q: The well-being of the relative or carer attending the patient is maintained Just being at the bedside can be a sign of support and caring. Consider spiritual/religious/cultural needs, expressions may be unfamiliar to the healthcare professional but normal for the relative or carer – support of chaplaincy team may be helpful. Listen & respond to worries/fears. Age appropriate advice & information to support children/adolescents available to parents or carers. Allow the opportunity to reminisce. Offer a drink						
Signature of the person making the assessment						
Signature of the registered nurse per shift	Night	Early		Late		Night

LCP generic version 12 – December 2009
© Marie Curie Palliative Care Institute Liverpool (MCPCIL)

ADD NAME OF ORGANISATION HERE

Name:... NHS no:... Date:...

Section 2   Ongoing assessment of the plan of care – LCP DAY........

Undertake an MDT assessment & review of the current management plan if:

| Improved conscious level, functional ability, oral intake, mobility, ability to perform self-care | **and or** | Concern expressed regarding management plan from either the patient, relative or team member | **and or** | It is 3 days since the last **full** MDT assessment |

Consider the support of the specialist palliative care team and/or a second opinion as required. Document all reassessment dates and times on page 3

Codes to be recorded at each timed assessment (a moment in time) A= Achieved V = Variance (exception reporting)

Record an A or a V not a signature	0400	0800	1200	1600	2000	2400
Goal a: The patient does not have pain Verbalised by patient if conscious, pain free on movement. Observe for non-verbal cues. Consider need for positional change. Use a pain assessment tool if appropriate. Consider prn analgesia for incident pain						
Goal b: The patient is not agitated Patient does not display signs of restlessness or distress, exclude reversible causes e.g. retention of urine, opioid toxicity						
Goal c: The patient does not have respiratory tract secretions Consider positional change. Discuss symptoms & plan of care with patient, relative or carer Medication to be given as soon as symptom occurs						
Goal d: The patient does not have nausea Verbalised by patient if conscious						
Goal e: The patient is not vomiting						
Goal f: The patient is not breathless Verbalised by patient if conscious, consider positional change. Use of a fan may be helpful						
Goal g: The patient does not have urinary problems Use of pads, urinary catheter as required						
Goal h: The patient does not have bowel problems Monitor – constipation / diarrhoea. Monitor skin integrity Bowels last opened:.........................						
Goal i: The patient does not have other symptoms Record symptom here... *If no other symptoms present please record N/A*						
Goal j: The patient's comfort & safety regarding the administration of medication is maintained If CSCI in place – monitoring sheet in progress S/C butterfly in place if needed for prn medication location:............................... The patient is only receiving medication that is beneficial at this time. *If no medication required please record N/A*						

LCP generic version 12 – December 2009
© Marie Curie Palliative Care Institute Liverpool (MCPCIL)

ADD NAME OF ORGANISATION HERE

Name:.. NHS no:.. Date:..................................

Section 2   Ongoing assessment of the plan of care – LCP continued DAY....

Codes to be recorded at each timed assessment (a moment in time) A= Achieved   V = Variance (exception reporting)

	0400	0800	1200	1600	2000	2400
Goal k: The patient receives fluids to support their individual needs The patient is supported to take oral fluids / thickened fluids for as long as tolerated. Monitor for signs of aspiration and/or distress. If symptomatically dehydrated & not deemed futile, consider clinically assisted (artificial) hydration if in the patient's best interest. If in place monitor & review rate/volume. Explain the plan of care with the patient and relative or carer						
Goal l: The patient's mouth is moist and clean See mouth care policy. Relative or carer involved in care giving as appropriate. Mouth care tray at the bedside						
Goal m: The patient's skin integrity is maintained Assessment, cleansing, positioning, use of special aids (mattress / bed). The frequency of repositioning should be determined by skin inspection and the patient's individual needs. *Waterlow / Braden score:*....................						
Goal n: The patient's personal hygiene needs are met Skin care, wash, eye care, change of clothing according to individual needs. Relative or carer involved in care giving as appropriate						
Goal o: The patient receives their care in a physical environment adjusted to support their individual needs Well fitting curtains, screens, clean environment, sufficient space at bedside, consider fragrance, silence, music, light, dark, pictures, photographs, nurse call bell accessible						
Goal p: The patient's psychological well-being is maintained Staff just being at the bedside can be a sign of support and caring. Respectful verbal and non-verbal communication, use of listening skills, information and explanation of care given. Use of touch if appropriate. Spiritual/religious/cultural needs – consider support of the chaplaincy team						
Goal q: The well-being of the relative or carer attending the patient is maintained Just being at the bedside can be a sign of support and caring. Consider spiritual/religious/cultural needs, expressions may be unfamiliar to the healthcare professional but normal for the relative or carer – support of chaplaincy team may be helpful. Listen & respond to worries/fears. Age appropriate advice & information to support children/adolescents available to parents or carers. Allow the opportunity to reminisce. Offer a drink						
Signature of the person making the assessment						
Signature of the registered nurse per shift	Night	Early		Late		Night

LCP generic version 12 – December 2009
© Marie Curie Palliative Care Institute Liverpool (MCPCIL)

ADD NAME OF ORGANISATION HERE

Name:.. NHS no:.. Date:

Section 2	Ongoing assessment MDT progress notes	
Date/time	Record significant events/conversations/medical review/visit by other specialist teams e.g. palliative care / second opinion if sought	Signature

Name:.. NHS no:..

Section 2	Ongoing assessment MDT progress notes	
Date / time	Record significant events/conversations/medical review/visit by other specialist teams e.g. palliative care/second opinion if sought	Signature

Name:.. NHS no:... Date:..

Section 3	Care after death

Verification of death

Time of the patient's death recorded by the healthcare professional in the organisation:...
Date of patient's death: ..../.........../.........
Verified by doctor ☐   Verified by senior nurse ☐   Date / time verified:..
Cause of death...

Details of healthcare professional who verified death
Name:.. (please print) Signature:..   Bleep No:........................
Comments:...
....
Persons present at time of death:...
Relative or carer present at time of death: Yes ☐ No ☐   If not present, have the relative or carer been notified Yes ☐ No ☐
Name of person informed:...   Relationship to the patient:...
Contact number:...
Is the coroner likely to be involved: Yes ☐ No ☐
Consultant /GP:...   Doctor:...................................   Bleep No:.............. Tel No:...................

Patient Care Dignity	**Goal 10: last offices are undertaken according to policy and procedure** Achieved ☐ Variance ☐ The patient is treated with respect and dignity whilst last offices are undertaken Universal precautions & local policy and procedures including infection risk adhered to Spiritual, religious, cultural rituals / needs met Organisational policy followed for the management of ICD's, where appropriate Organisational policy followed for the management & storage of patient's valuables and belongings
Relative or Carer Information	**Goal 11: The relative or carer can express an understanding of what they will need to do next and are given relevant written information** Achieved ☐ Variance ☐ Conversation with relative or carer explaining the next steps Grieving leaflet given Yes ☐ No ☐ DWP1027 (England & Wales) or equivalent is given Yes ☐ No ☐ Information given regarding how and when to contact the bereavement office / general office / funeral director to make an appointment – regarding the death certificate and patient's valuables and belongings where appropriate Wishes regarding tissue/organ donation discussed Discuss as appropriate: viewing the body / the need for a post mortem / the need for removal of cardiac devices / the need for a discussion with the coroner Information given to families on child bereavement services where appropriate – national & local agencies
Organisation Information	**Goal 12.1: The primary health care team / GP is notified of the patient's death** Achieved ☐ Variance ☐ The primary health care team / GP may have known this patient very well and other relatives or carers may be registered with the same GP. Telephone or fax the GP practice **Goal 12.2: The patient's death is communicated to appropriate services across the organisation** Achieved ☐ Variance ☐ e.g. Bereavement office / general office / palliative care team / district nursing team / community matron (where appropriate) are informed of the death The patient's death is entered on the organisations IT system

Healthcare professional signature:...
Date:..   **Time:**...

Please record any variance on the variance sheet overleaf

Section 3   Care after death MDT progress notes   - *record any significant issues not reflected above*

Date	

LCP generic version 12 – December 2009   ADD NAME OF ORGANISATION HERE
© Marie Curie Palliative Care Institute Liverpool (MCPCIL)

Name:.. NHS no:.. Date:..

Variance analysis sheet for section 2 and 3 of the LCP		
What variance occurred & why? (what was the issue?)	Action taken (what did you do?)	Outcome (did this solve the issue?)
Goal: Signature:.. Date / Time:.....................................	 Signature:.. Date / Time:.....................................	 Signature:.. Date / Time:.....................................
Goal: Signature:.. Date / Time:.....................................	 Signature:.. Date / Time:.....................................	 Signature:.. Date / Time:.....................................
Goal: Signature:.. Date / Time:.....................................	 Signature:.. Date / Time:.....................................	 Signature:.. Date / Time:.....................................
Goal: Signature:.. Date / Time:.....................................	 Signature:.. Date / Time:.....................................	 Signature:.. Date / Time:.....................................
Goal: Signature:.. Date / Time:.....................................	 Signature:.. Date / Time:.....................................	 Signature:.. Date / Time:.....................................

LCP generic version 12 – December 2009
© Marie Curie Palliative Care Institute Liverpool (MCPCIL)

ADD NAME OF ORGANISATION HERE

LCP supporting information

All documents/leaflets listed below can be viewed and ordered via our Marie Curie Palliative Care Institute Liverpool website http://www.mcpcil.org.uk

- **Relative & Carer LCP information leaflet** www.mcpcil.org.uk

- **Healthcare professional LCP information** www.mcpcil.org.uk

- **Medication guidance - See an example of a locally designed medication guidance document at:** www.mcpcil.org.uk
  Each organisation should produce their own medication guidance in support of the LCP in accordance to local medicine management group, policy/procedures in liaison with specialist palliative care colleagues

- **Facilities leaflet - Organisations need to design their own leaflet to reflect local facilities within the environment** Content may include - car parking, public transport, refreshments, cash machine. pay phone, accommodation, chaplaincy support

- **Coping with dying leaflet** www.mcpcil.org.uk

- **Grieving leaflet - Organisations need to design their own leaflet to reflect local service availability within the environment and health economy** Content may include what does grieving feel like, things to consider, signposting to local & national organisations

- **Helpful references document** http://www.mcpcil.org.uk/liverpool-care-pathway/research.htm

- **LCP supporting information customer order form** www.mcpcil.org.uk

- **Example of section 2 ongoing assessment sheet for a non inpatient setting, where registered (trained) nursing care is not available 24 hrs per day** e.g. patient's own home or residential care / community setting www.mcpcil.org.uk

Appendix 2

Section 2   Ongoing assessment of the plan of care – LCP DAY........

Undertake an MDT assessment & review of the current management plan if:

Improved conscious level, functional ability, oral intake, mobility, ability to perform self-care	and/ or	Concern expressed regarding management plan from either the patient, relative or team member	and/ or	It is 3 days since the last **full** MDT assessment

Consider the support of the specialist palliative care team and/or second opinion as required. Document all reassessment dates and times on page 3

Codes to be recorded at each timed assessment (a moment in time)   A= Achieved   V = Variance (exception reporting)

Record an A or a V not a signature

Date/Time per visit						
Goal a: The patient does not have pain Verbalised by patient if conscious, pain free on movement. Observe for non-verbal cues. Consider need for positional change. Use a pain assessment tool if appropriate. Consider prn analgesia for incident pain						
Goal b: The patient is not agitated Patient does not display signs of restlessness or distress, exclude reversible causes e.g. retention of urine, opioid toxicity						
Goal c: The patient does not have respiratory tract secretions Consider positional change. Discuss symptoms & plan of care with patient, relative or carer Medication to be given as soon as symptom occurs						
Goal d: The patient does not have nausea Verbalised by patient if conscious						
Goal e: The patient is not vomiting						
Goal f: The patient is not breathless Verbalised by patient if conscious, consider positional change. Use of a fan may be helpful						
Goal g: The patient does not have urinary problems Use of pads, urinary catheter as required						
Goal h: The patient does not have bowel problems Monitor – constipation / diarrhoea. Monitor skin integrity Bowels last opened:..........................						
Goal i: The patient does not have other symptoms Record symptom here... *If no other symptoms present please record N/A*						
Goal j: The patient's comfort & safety regarding the administration of medication is maintained If CSCI in place – monitoring sheet in progress S/C butterfly in place if needed for prn medication location:............................. The patient is only receiving medication that is beneficial at this time. *If no medication required please record N/A*						

> **Example of Section 2 Ongoing assessment sheet for a non inpatient setting, where registered (trained) nursing care is not available 24 hrs per day e.g. patient's own home or residential care / community setting**

Section 2   Ongoing assessment of the plan of care – LCP continued DAY....

Codes to be recorded at each timed assessment (a moment in time) A= Achieved   V = Variance (exception reporting)

Date/Time per visit						
Goal k: The patient receives fluids to support their individual needs The patient is supported to take oral fluids / thickened fluids for as long as tolerated. Monitor for signs of aspiration and/or distress. If symptomatically dehydrated & not deemed futile, consider clinically assisted (artificial) hydration if in the patient's best interest. If in place monitor & review rate/volume. Explain the plan of care with the patient and relative or carer						
Goal l: The patient's mouth is moist and clean See mouth care policy. Relative or carer involved in care giving as appropriate. Mouth care tray at the bedside.						
Goal m: The patient's skin integrity is maintained Assessment, cleansing, positioning, use of special aids (mattress / bed). The frequency of repositioning should be determined by skin inspection and the patient's individual needs. *Waterlow / Braden score:.....................*						
Goal n: The patient's personal hygiene needs are met Skin care, wash, eye care, change of clothing according to individual needs. Relative or carer involved in care giving as appropriate						
Goal o: The patient receives their care in a physical environment adjusted to support their individual needs Well fitting curtains, screens, clean environment, sufficient space at bedside, consider fragrance, silence/music, light/dark, pictures/photographs, nurse call bell accessible						
Goal p: The patient's psychological well-being is maintained Staff just being at the bedside can be a sign of support and caring. Respectful verbal and non-verbal communication, use of listening skills, information and explanation of care given. Use of touch if appropriate. Spiritual/religious/cultural needs – consider support of the chaplaincy team						
Goal q: The well-being of the relative or carer attending the patient is maintained Just being at the bedside can be a sign of support and caring. Consider spiritual/religious/cultural needs, expressions may be unfamiliar to the healthcare professional but normal for the relative or carer – support of chaplaincy team may be helpful. Listen & respond to worries/fears. Age appropriate advice & information to support children/adolescents available to parents or carers. Allow the opportunity to reminisce. Offer/provide a drink						
Signature of the person making the assessment						
Signature of the registered nurse per visit						

ADD NAME OF ORGANISATION HERE

Appendix 3

 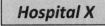 1

Name *Karen Jackson*　　　　NHS no *9998887777*　　　　Date *05.04.10*

Liverpool Care Pathway for the Dying Patient (LCP)
supporting care in the last hours or days of life

Ward: 2F

As with all clinical guidelines and pathways the LCP aims to support but does not replace clinical judgement

- ❑ The LCP generic document guides and enables healthcare professionals to focus on care in the last hours or days of life. This provides high quality care tailored to the patient's individual needs, when their death is expected.

- ❑ Using the LCP in any environment requires regular assessment and involves regular reflection, challenge, critical senior decision-making and clinical skill, in the best interest of the patient. A robust continuous learning and teaching programme must underpin the use of the LCP.

- ❑ The recognition and diagnosis of dying is always complex; irrespective of previous diagnosis or history. Uncertainty is an integral part of dying. There are occasions when a patient who is thought to be dying lives longer than expected and vice versa. Seek a second opinion or specialist palliative care support as needed.

- ❑ Changes in care at this complex, uncertain time are made in the best interest of the patient and relative or carer and needs to be reviewed regularly by the multidisciplinary team (MDT).

- ❑ Good comprehensive clear communication is pivotal and all decisions leading to a change in care delivery should be communicated to the patient where appropriate and to the relative or carer. The views of all concerned must be listened to and documented.

- ❑ If a goal on the LCP is not achieved this should be coded as a variance. This is not a negative process but demonstrates the individual nature of the patient's condition based on their particular needs, your clinical judgement and the needs of the relative or carer.

- ❑ The LCP does not preclude the use of clinically assisted nutrition or hydration or antibiotics. All clinical decisions must be made in the patient's best interest.

- ❑ A blanket policy of clinically assisted (artificial) nutrition or hydration, or of no clinically assisted (artificial) hydration, is ethically indefensible and in the case of patients lacking capacity prohibited under the Mental Capacity Act (2005).

- ❑ For the purpose of this LCP generic version 12 document - The term best interest includes medical, physical, emotional, social and spiritual and all other factors relevant to the patient's welfare.

The patient will be assessed regularly and a formal full MDT review must be undertaken every 3 days.

The responsibility for the use of the LCP generic document as part of a continuous quality improvement programme sits within the governance of an organisation and must be underpinned by a robust education and training programme.

References:
Ellershaw, J. & Wilkinson, S. (eds) (2011) *Care of the dying: a pathway to excellence*. 2nd ed. Oxford: Oxford University Press.
National Institute for Clinical Excellence (2004) Improving Supportive and Palliative Care for Adults with Cancer. London, NICE
MCPCIL (2009) National Care of the Dying Audit Hospitals Generic Report Round 2. www.mcpcil.org.uk
Merseyside and Cheshire Palliative Care Network Audit Group (2009) Standards and Guidelines Fourth Edition.

Name **Karen Jackson**   NHS no **9998887777**   Date **05.04.10**

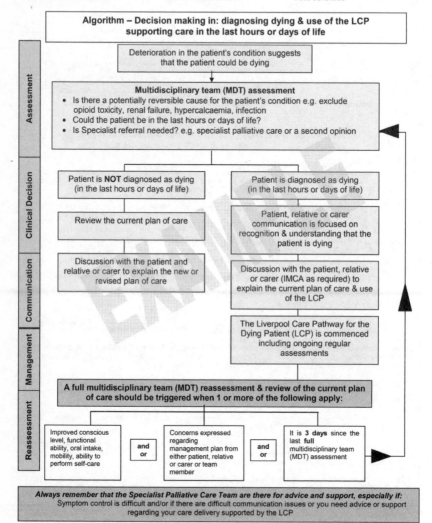

LCP generic version 12 – April 2010
© Marie Curie Palliative Care Institute Liverpool (MCPCIL)

Hospital X

Name **Karen Jackson** NHS no **9998887777** Date **05.04.10**

Healthcare professional documenting the MDT decision
Following a full MDT assessment and a decision to use the LCP:

Date LCP commenced: 05/04/10

Time LCP commenced: 15:35

Name (Print): DR J JONES (SPR) **Signature:** *J Jones*

This should be the most senior healthcare professional immediately available, i.e. Consultant or StR (Specialist Trainee Registrar)

The decision must be endorsed by the most senior healthcare professional responsible for the patient's care at the earliest opportunity if different from above, i.e. Consultant

Name (Print): DR. WILLIAM HARRISON (Consultant) Signature: *W. Harrison* 06.04.10

All personnel completing the LCP please sign below
You should also have read and understood the guidance on pages 1 - 2

Name (print)	Full signature	Initials	Professional title	Date
DR J JONES	*J Jones*	JJ	SPR	05/04/10
DR A SMITH	**A.SMITH**	AS	F1	05/04/10
KELLY BARR	Kelly Barr	KB	RGN	05/04/10
MICHELLE COOPER	M. COOPER	MC	Palliative Care Nurse	05/04/10
RACHEL DOYLE	Rachel Doyle	RD	RGN	05/04/10
PHIL SULLIVAN	P. Sullivan	PS	RGN	06/04/10
DR. S. HUGHES	**S Hughes**	**SH**	**F2**	**06/04/10**
A. PRICE	A Price	AP	Palliative Care CNS	7/4/10
L ROBERTS	L. Roberts	LR	RGN	07/04/10
Fr. M. Williams	Michael Williams	MW	Priest RC	08/04/10

Record all full MDT reassessments here (including full formal MDT reassessment every 3 days)

Reassessment date: **7/4/10** Reassessment time: **10.00hrs – Ward round:**

Reassessment date:... Reassessment time:...

Reassessment date:... Reassessment time:...

Reassessment date:... Reassessment time:...

If the LCP is discontinued please record here:

Date LCP discontinued................................. Time LCP discontinued.................................

Reasons why the LCP was discontinued:...

....

....

Decision to discontinue the LCP shared with the patient **Yes ☐ No ☐**

Decision to discontinue the LCP shared with the relative or carer **Yes ☐ No ☐**

Name *Karen Jackson*   NHS no *9998887777*   Date *05.04.10*

Section 1	Initial assessment (joint assessment by doctor and nurse)

DIAGNOSIS: Bowel Cancer   Co-morbidity: /
Ethnicity: White / British   DOB: 10.06.1963   Age: 46   NHS no: 9998887777

Female ☑ Male ☐

At the time of the assessment is the patient:

In pain	Yes ☑ No☐	Able to swallow	Yes ☑ No ☐	Confused	Yes ☐ No ☑
Agitated	Yes ☐ No ☑	Continent (bladder)	Yes ☑ No ☐	*(record below which is applicable)*	
Nauseated	Yes ☐ No ☑	Catheterised	Yes ☑ No ☐	Conscious	☑
Vomiting	Yes ☐ No ☑	Continent (bowels)	Yes ☑ No ☐	Semi-conscious	☐
Dyspnoeic	Yes ☐ No ☑	Constipated	Yes ☐ No ☑	Unconscious	☐
Experiencing respiratory tract secretions			Yes ☐ No ☑		
Experiencing other symptoms (e.g. oedema, itch)			Yes ☐ No ☑		

Diagnosis & Baseline Information

Goal 1.1: The patient is able to take a full and active part in communication

Achieved ☑ Variance ☐ Unconscious ☐

Barriers that have the potential to prevent communication have been assessed
First language English   Other issues identified ...../ ....
Consider need for an interpreter: (contact no) ..../ ....
Other barriers to communication................/ ....
Consider: Hearing, vision, speech, learning disabilities, dementia (use of assessment tools), neurological conditions and confusion
The relative or carer may know how specific signs indicate distress if the patient is unable to articulate their own concerns
Does the patient have:-
An advance care plan?
An expressed wish for organ/tissue donation?
An advance decision to refuse treatment (ADRT)?
Does the patient have the capacity to make their own decisions on their own treatment at this moment in time?
consider the support of an IMCA – if required document below:
Comments:.../ ....

Goal 1.2:   The relative or carer is able to take a full and active part in communication   Achieved ☑   Variance ☐
First language English   Other Issues identified....../ ....
Consider need for an interpreter (contact no):...../ ....
Other barriers to communication:.../ ....

Goal 1.3:   The patient is aware that they are dying   Achieved ☑ Variance ☐ Unconscious ☐

Goal 1.4:   The relative or carer is aware that the patient is dying   Achieved ☑ Variance ☐

Goal 1.5:   The Clinical team have up to date contact information for the relative or carer as documented below

Achieved ☑   Variance ☐

1st contact name: Bob Jackson
Relationship to the patient: Husband   Tel no: **0012 123 0037**   Mobile no: **03344668810**
When to contact: At any time☐   Not at night-time ☐   Staying with the patient overnight ☑

2nd contact: Elizabeth Jackson

Relationship to the patient: Sister-in-law   Tel no: 222-3333   Mobile no:..../ ....
When to contact: At any time ☑   Not at night-time ☐   Staying with the patient overnight ☐

Next of kin - this may be different from above N/A ☑	**Lasting Power of Attorney (LPA) (if applicable)** N/A ☑
Name:........ /	Name:...... / ....
Contact details:..... /	Contact details:..... / ....

Communication

Name **Karen Jackson**   NHS no 9998887777   Date **05.04.10**

Section 1	Initial assessment (joint assessment by doctor and nurse)

Facilities

Goal 2:The relative or carer has had a full explanation of the facilities available to them and a facilities leaflet has been given   Achieved ☑   Variance ☐

Facilities may include: car parking, toilet, bathroom facilities, beverages, payphone, accommodation
Facilities leaflet available in the LCP box file located on each ward

Spirituality

Goal 3.1:   The patient is given the opportunity to discuss what is important to them at this time eg. their wishes, feelings, faith , beliefs, values   Achieved ☑   Variance ☐   Unconscious ☐
Patient may be anxious for self or others. Consider specific religious and cultural needs
Consider music, art, poetry, reading, photographs, something that has been important to the belief system or the well-being of the patient

Did the patient take the opportunity to discuss the above   Yes ☑ No ☐ Unconscious ☐
Religious tradition identified, please specify: R/C
Support of the chaplaincy team offered   Yes ☑ No ☐
If no give reason:
In-house support   Tel/bleep no: ...../ .... Name: ..../ .... Date/time: .../ ....
External support   Tel/bleep no: ...../ .... Name: ..../ .... Date/time: .../ ....

Needs now: No specific needs now – requested not to be seen by a priest

Needs at death: Karen wants to be seen by a priest at death

Needs after death: no specific needs identified – R/C religious tradition

Goal 3.2:   The relative or carer is given the opportunity to discuss what is important to them at this time e.g. their wishes, feelings, faith, beliefs, values   Achieved ☑   Variance ☐
Comments: Pastoral care / Chaplaincy information leaflet given to Mr. Jackson – family photograph at the bedside

Did the relative or carer take the opportunity to discuss the above   Yes ☑   No ☐

Medication

Goal 4.1:   The patient has medication prescribed on a prn basis for all of the following 5 symptoms which may develop in the last hours or days of life   Achieved ☑   Variance ☐
Pain   ☑
Agitation   ☑
Respiratory tract secretions   ☑
Nausea / Vomiting   ☑
Dyspnoea   ☑

Anticipatory prescribing in this manner will ensure that there is no delay in responding to a symptom if it occurs
Current Medication assessed and non essentials discontinued. See drug guidance page 20-22
Medicines for symptom control will only be given when needed, at the right time and just enough and no more than is needed to help the symptom

Goal 4.2: Equipment is available for the patient to support a continuous subcutaneous infusion (CSCI) of medication where required
          Achieved ☐   Variance ☐   Already in place ☐   Not required ☑
If a CSCI is to be used explain the rationale to the patient, relative or carer. Not all patients who are dying will require a CSCI

Name **Karen Jackson**   NHS no 9998887777   Date **05.04.10**

Section 1	Initial assessment (joint assessment by doctor and nurse)

Current Interventions

Goal 5.1: The patient's need for current interventions has been reviewed by the MDT   Achieved ☐ Variance ☐

		Currently not being taken/ or given	Discontinued	Continued	Commenced
5a:	Routine blood tests	☐	☑	☐	
5b:	Intravenous antibiotics	☑	☐	☐	☐
5c:	Blood glucose monitoring	☑	☐	☐	
5d:	Recording of routine vital signs	☐	☑	☐	
5e:	Oxygen therapy	☑	☐	☐	☐

5.2: The patient has a Do Not Attempt Cardiopulmonary Resuscitation Order in place   Achieved ☑ Variance ☐
Please complete the associated documentation (red card) according to policy and procedure
Explain to the patient, relative or carer as appropriate

5.3: Implantable Cardioverter Defibrillator (ICD) is deactivated   Achieved ☐ Variance ☐ No ICD in place ☑
Contact the patient's cardiologist. Refer to the ECG technician & refer to local/ regional - policy/procedure.
Information leaflet given to the patient, relative or carer as appropriate

Nutrition

Goal 6: The need for clinically assisted (artificial) nutrition is reviewed by the MDT   Achieved ☑ Variance ☐
The patient should be supported to take food by mouth for as long as tolerated
For many patients the use of clinically assisted (artificial) nutrition will not be required
A reduced need for food is part of the normal dying process
If clinically assisted (artificial) nutrition is already in place please record route   NG ☐   PEG/PEJ ☐   NJ ☐   TPN ☐
Is clinically assisted (artificial) nutrition   Not required ☑ Discontinued ☐   Continued ☐
Consider reduction in rate / volume according to individual need if nutritional support is in place
Explain the plan of care to the patient where appropriate, and to the relative or carer

Hydration

Goal 7: The need for clinically assisted (artificial) hydration is reviewed by the MDT   Achieved ☑ Variance ☐
The patient should be supported to take fluids by mouth for as long as tolerated
For many patients the use of clinically assisted (artificial) hydration will not be required
A reduced need for fluids is part of the normal dying process
Symptoms of thirst / dry mouth do not always indicate dehydration but are often due to mouth breathing or medication. Good mouth care is essential
If clinically assisted (artificial) hydration is already in place please record route   IV ☑   S/C ☐ PEG/PEJ ☐   NG ☐
Is clinically assisted (artificial) hydration   Not required ☐   Discontinued ☐   Continued ☑   Commenced ☐
Consider reduction in rate / volume according to individual need if hydration support is in place. If required consider the s/c route
Explain the plan of care to the patient where appropriate, and the relative or carer

Skin Care

Goal 8: The patient's skin integrity is assessed   Achieved ☑ Variance ☐
The aim is to prevent pressure ulcers or further deterioration if a pressure ulcer is present. Use a recognised risk assessment tool
e.g. Waterlow to support clinical judgement. The frequency of repositioning should be determined by skin inspection, assessment
and the patient's individual needs. Consider the use of special aids (mattress / bed)
Record the plan of care on the initial assessment MDT sheet where appropriate

Explanation of the plan of care

Goal 9.1: A full explanation of the current plan of care (LCP) is given to the patient
                                                      Achieved ☑ Variance ☐ Unconscious ☐

Goal 9.2: A full explanation of the current plan of care (LCP) is given to the relative or carer
                                                      Achieved ☑ Variance ☐
Name of relative or carer(s) present and relationship to the patient: Bob Jackson (Husband)
Names of healthcare professionals present: K.Barr (RGN)
Information sheet at front of the LCP or equivalent relative or carer information leaflet given   Yes ☑ No ☐
Parents or carer should be given or have access to age appropriate advice and information to support children/adolescents

Goal 9.3: The LCP Coping with dying leaflet or equivalent is given to the relative or carer
                                                      Achieved ☑ Variance ☐
Coping with dying leaflet available in the LCP box file located in each ward

Goal 9.4: The patient's primary health care team / GP practice is notified that the patient is dying
                                                      Achieved ☑ Variance ☐
G.P practice to be contacted if unaware that the patient is dying, message can be left or sent via a secure fax

If you have recorded a variance against any of the goals of care please record on the variance sheet, see page 8

Name **Karen Jackson**   NHS **9998887777**   Date **05.04.10**

Section 1	Initial assessment

Please sign here on completion of the initial assessment

<table>
<tr><td rowspan="4">Signatures</td><td>Doctor's name (print): DR A SMITH (F1)</td><td>Nurse's name (print): KELLY BARR</td></tr>
<tr><td>Doctor's signature: A.SMITH</td><td>Nurse's signature: Kelly Barr</td></tr>
<tr><td>(F1, F2, StR, Consultant)</td><td>Registered Nurse</td></tr>
<tr><td>Date 5/4/10   Time 15:40</td><td>Date 05/04/10   Time15:40</td></tr>
</table>

Section 1	Initial assessment MDT progress notes

Date	Supportive information: Plan of care to monitor skin integrity, nutrition / hydration - include here any specific information regarding this patient; relative or carer that has not been captured in the initial assessment that you believe needs to be highlighted.
05.04.10	Following a long discussion with Karen and her husband, Mr. Jackson has gone home to speak with their
1540	adult children aged 18, 20, 22. Please call the palliative care department on extension 3014 when Mr.
	Jackson (Karen's Husband) and children are on the ward and the palliative care nurse specialist will review.
	<div align="right">Kelly Barr (RGN)</div>
05.04.10	*Palliative Care Team*
1645 Hours	*Thank you, I met with the patient, her husband and their 3 children, Emma, James and Jonathon. Also spoke to*
	the children separately. Very upset but understand the current plan of care and very happy with ward care delivery.
	We will continue to review. I will review again in the morning. Out of Hours support number made available to
	the staff on the ward should this be required. / family aware of Out of Hours advice line
	<div align="right">*M. Cooper*</div>
	<div align="right">*Palliative Care Nurse*</div>
	<div align="right">*Ext. 3014 Bleep 1122*</div>
05.04.10	Mr. Jackson (husband) and his 3 children seen by the palliative care nurse specialist, fully aware of current plan.
1700	All staying with Karen overnight.
	<div align="right">Kelly Barr (RGN)</div>

Name *Karen Jackson*   NHS *9998887777*   Date *05.04.10*

Variance analysis sheet for section 1 - initial assessment

What variance occurred & why? (What was the issue?)	Action taken (What did you do?)	Outcome (Did this solve the issue?)
Goal: Patient in pain *Signature:* Kelly Barr *Date / Time:* 5.4.10 1540 hours	Following an assessment, morphine 5mgs given s/c. Review in 20 minutes *Signature:* Kelly Barr *Date / Time:* 5.4.10 1545 hours	Patient reviewed, pain now settled, review again in 1 hour. *Signature:* Kelly Barr *Date / Time:* 5.4.10 1600 hours
Goal: Relatives and patient asking for IV hydration to continue but venflon site inflamed *Signature:* Kelly Barr *Date / Time:* 5.4.10 1545 hours	S/C fluids in place – 1 litre in 24 hours *Signature:* Kelly Barr *Date / Time:* 5.4.10 1545 hours	I reviewed patient and met with relatives – happy with s/c fluids – situation to be monitor. Site dry and intact *Signature:* Kelly Barr *Date / Time:* 5.4.10 1615 hours
Goal: *Signature:*........................... *Date / Time:*...........................	*Signature:*........................... *Date / Time:*...........................	*Signature:*........................... *Date / Time:*...........................
Goal: *Signature:*........................... *Date / Time:*...........................	*Signature:*........................... *Date / Time:*...........................	*Signature:*........................... *Date / Time:*...........................
Goal: *Signature:*........................... *Date / Time:*...........................	*Signature:*........................... *Date / Time:*...........................	*Signature:*........................... *Date / Time:*...........................

Name **Karen Jackson**   NHS **9998887777**   Date **05.04.10**

Section 2   Ongoing assessment of the plan of care – LCP DAY 1

Undertake an MDT assessment & review of the current management plan if:

Improved conscious level, functional ability, oral intake, mobility, ability to perform self-care	and or	Concern expressed regarding management plan from either the patient, relative or team member	and or	It is 3 days since the last **full** MDT assessment

Consider the support of the specialist palliative care team and/or a second opinion as required. Document all reassessment dates and times on page 3

Codes to be recorded at each timed assessment (a moment in time)   A= Achieved   V = Variance (exception reporting)

Record an A or a V not a signature	0400	0800	1200	1600	2000	2400
Goal a: The patient does not have pain Verbalised by patient if conscious, pain free on movement. Observe for non-verbal cues. Consider need for positional change. Use a pain assessment tool if appropriate. Consider prn analgesia for incident pain	/	/	/	A	A	V
Goal b: The patient is not agitated Patient does not display signs of restlessness or distress, exclude reversible causes e.g. retention of urine, opioid toxicity	/	/	/	A	A	A
Goal c: The patient does not have respiratory tract secretions Consider positional change. Discuss symptoms & plan of care with patient, relative or carer Medication to be given as soon as symptom occurs	/	/	/	A	A	A
Goal d: The patient does not have nausea Verbalised by patient if conscious	/	/	/	A	A	A
Goal e: The patient is not vomiting	/	/	/	A	A	A
Goal f: The patient is not breathless Verbalised by patient if conscious, consider positional change. Use of a fan may be helpful	/	/	/	A	A	A
Goal g: The patient does not have urinary problems Use of pads, urinary catheter as required	/	/	/	A	A	A
Goal h: The patient does not have bowel problems Monitor – constipation / diarrhoea. Monitor skin integrity Bowels last opened: 04.04.10	/	/	/	A	A	A
Goal i: The patient does not have other symptoms Record symptom here Pruritus (itch) *If no other symptoms present please record N/A*	/	/	/	A	A	A
Goal j: The patient's comfort & safety regarding the administration of medication is maintained If CSCI in place – monitoring sheet in progress S/C butterfly in place if needed for prn medication location:.............................. The patient is only receiving medication that is beneficial at this time. *If no medication required please record N/A*	/	/	/	A	A	A

LCP generic version 12 – April 2010   Hospital X
© Marie Curie Palliative Care Institute Liverpool (MCPCIL)

Name **Karen Jackson**   NHS **9998887777**   Date **05.04.10**

Section 2   Ongoing assessment of the plan of care – LCP DAY / continued

Codes to be recorded at each timed assessment (a moment in time) A= Achieved   V = Variance (exception reporting)

	0400	0800	1200	1600	2000	2400
Goal k: The patient receives fluids to support their individual needs The patient is supported to take oral fluids / thickened fluids for as long as tolerated. Monitor for signs of aspiration and/or distress. If symptomatically dehydrated & not deemed futile, consider clinically assisted (artificial) hydration if in the patient's best interest. If in place monitor & review rate/volume. Explain the plan of care with the patient and relative or carer	/	/	/	A	A	V
Goal l: The patient's mouth is moist and clean See mouth care policy. Relative or carer involved in care giving as appropriate. Mouth care tray at the bedside	/	/	/	A	A	A
Goal m: The patient's skin integrity is maintained Assessment, cleansing, positioning, use of special aids (mattress / bed). The frequency of repositioning should be determined by skin inspection and the patient's individual needs. *Waterlow score:*..................	/	/	/	A	A	A
Goal n: The patient's personal hygiene needs are met Skin care, wash, eye care, change of clothing according to individual needs. Relative or carer involved in care giving as appropriate	/	/	/	A	A	A
Goal o: The patient receives their care in a physical environment adjusted to support their individual needs Well fitting curtains, screens, clean environment, sufficient space at bedside, consider fragrance, silence, music, light, dark, pictures, photographs, nurse call bell accessible	/	/	/	A	A	A
Goal p: The patient's psychological well-being is maintained Staff just being at the bedside can be a sign of support and caring. Respectful verbal and non-verbal communication, use of listening skills, information and explanation of care given. Use of touch if appropriate. Spiritual/religious/cultural needs – consider support of the chaplaincy team	/	/	/	A	A	A
Goal q: The well-being of the relative or carer attending the patient is maintained Just being at the bedside can be a sign of support and caring. Consider spiritual/religious/cultural needs, expressions may be unfamiliar to the healthcare professional but normal for the relative or carer – support of chaplaincy team may be helpful. Listen & respond to worries/fears. Age appropriate advice & information to support children/adolescents available to parents or carers. Allow the opportunity to reminisce. Offer a drink	/	/	/	A	A	A
Signature of the person making the assessment				K Barr	K Barr	R. Doyle
Signature of the registered nurse per shift	Night	Early		Late K. Barr		Night R. Doyle

LCP generic version 12 – April 2010   Hospital X
© Marie Curie Palliative Care Institute Liverpool (MCPCIL)

Name **Karen Jackson**   NHS no 9998887777   Date 06.04.10

Section 2   Ongoing assessment of the plan of care – LCP DAY 2

Undertake an MDT assessment & review of the current management plan if:

Improved conscious level, functional ability, oral intake, mobility, ability to perform self-care	**and** **or**	Concern expressed regarding management plan from either the patient, relative or team member	**and** **or**	It is 3 days since the last **full** MDT assessment

Consider the support of the specialist palliative care team and/or a second opinion as required. Document all reassessment dates and times on page 3

Codes to be recorded at each timed assessment (a moment in time)   A= Achieved   V = Variance (exception reporting)

Record an A or a V not a signature	0400	0800	1200	1600	2000	2400
Goal a: The patient does not have pain Verbalised by patient if conscious, pain free on movement. Observe for non-verbal cues. Consider need for positional change. Use a pain assessment tool if appropriate. Consider prn analgesia for incident pain	A	A	A	A	A	A
Goal b: The patient is not agitated Patient does not display signs of restlessness or distress, exclude reversible causes e.g. retention of urine, opioid toxicity	A	A	A	A	A	A
Goal c: The patient does not have respiratory tract secretions Consider positional change. Discuss symptoms & plan of care with patient, relative or carer Medication to be given as soon as symptom occurs	A	A	A	A	A	A
Goal d: The patient does not have nausea Verbalised by patient if conscious	A	A	A	A	A	A
Goal e: The patient is not vomiting	A	A	A	A	A	A
Goal f: The patient is not breathless Verbalised by patient if conscious, consider positional change. Use of a fan may be helpful	A	A	A	A	A	A
Goal g: The patient does not have urinary problems Use of pads, urinary catheter as required	A	A	A	A	A	A
Goal h: The patient does not have bowel problems Monitor – constipation / diarrhoea. Monitor skin integrity Bowels last opened:4.04.10	A	A	A	A	A	A
Goal i: The patient does not have other symptoms Record symptom here Pruritus *If no other symptoms present please record N/A*	A	A	A	A	A	A
Goal j: The patient's comfort & safety regarding the administration of medication is maintained If CSCI in place – monitoring sheet in progress S/C butterfly in place if needed for prn medication location:.............................. The patient is only receiving medication that is beneficial at this time. *If no medication required please record N/A*	A	A	A	A	A	A

Name **Karen Jackson**   NHS no **9998887777**   Date **06.04.10**

Section 2   Ongoing assessment of the plan of care – LCP DAY 2 continued

Codes to be recorded at each timed assessment (a moment in time) A= Achieved   V = Variance (exception reporting)

	0400	0800	1200	1600	2000	2400
Goal k: The patient receives fluids to support their individual needs The patient is supported to take oral fluids / thickened fluids for as long as tolerated. Monitor for signs of aspiration and/or distress. If symptomatically dehydrated & not deemed futile, consider clinically assisted (artificial) hydration if in the patient's best interest. If in place monitor & review rate/volume. Explain the plan of care with the patient and relative or carer	V	A	A	A	A	A
Goal l: The patient's mouth is moist and clean See mouth care policy. Relative or carer involved in care giving as appropriate. Mouth care tray at the bedside	A	A	A	A	A	A
Goal m: The patient's skin integrity is maintained Assessment, cleansing, positioning, use of special aids (mattress / bed). The frequency of repositioning should be determined by skin inspection and the patient's individual needs. *Waterlow score:....................*	A	A	A	A	A	A
Goal n: The patient's personal hygiene needs are met Skin care, wash, eye care, change of clothing according to individual needs. Relative or carer involved in care giving as appropriate	A	A	A	A	A	A
Goal o: The patient receives their care in a physical environment adjusted to support their individual needs Well fitting curtains, screens, clean environment, sufficient space at bedside, consider fragrance, silence, music, light, dark, pictures, photographs, nurse call bell accessible	A	A	A	A	A	A
Goal p: The patient's psychological well-being is maintained Staff just being at the bedside can be a sign of support and caring. Respectful verbal and non-verbal communication, use of listening skills, information and explanation of care given. Use of touch if appropriate. Spiritual/religious/cultural needs – consider support of the chaplaincy team	A	A	A	A	A	A
Goal q: The well-being of the relative or carer attending the patient is maintained Just being at the bedside can be a sign of support and caring. Consider spiritual/religious/cultural needs, expressions may be unfamiliar to the healthcare professional but normal for the relative or carer – support of chaplaincy team may be helpful. Listen & respond to worries/fears. Age appropriate advice & information to support children/adolescents available to parents or carers. Allow the opportunity to reminisce. Offer a drink	A	A	A	A	A	A
Signature of the person making the assessment	R. Doyle	K Barr	K Barr	K Barr	K Barr	P Sullivan
Signature of the registered nurse per shift	**Night** R. Doyle	**Early** K Barr		**Late** K Barr		**Night** P Sullivan

LCP generic version 12 – April 2010
© Marie Curie Palliative Care Institute Liverpool (MCPCIL)

Hospital X

Name **Karen Jackson**   NHS no **9998887777**   Date 07.04.10

Section 2   Ongoing assessment of the plan of care – LCP DAY 3

Undertake an MDT assessment & review of the current management plan if:

| Improved conscious level, functional ability, oral intake, mobility, ability to perform self-care | and / or | Concern expressed regarding management plan from either the patient, relative or team member | and / or | It is 3 days since the last **full** MDT assessment |

Consider the support of the specialist palliative care team and/or a second opinion as required. Document all reassessment dates and times on page 3

Codes to be recorded at each timed assessment (a moment in time)   A= Achieved   V = Variance (exception reporting)

Record an A or a V not a signature	0400	0800	1200	1600	2000	2400
Goal a: The patient does not have pain Verbalised by patient if conscious, pain free on movement. Observe for non-verbal cues. Consider need for positional change. Use a pain assessment tool if appropriate. Consider prn analgesia for incident pain	A	A	A	A	A	A
Goal b: The patient is not agitated Patient does not display signs of restlessness or distress, exclude reversible causes e.g. retention of urine, opioid toxicity	A	A	A	A	A	A
Goal c: The patient does not have respiratory tract secretions Consider positional change. Discuss symptoms & plan of care with patient, relative or carer Medication to be given as soon as symptom occurs	A	A	A	A	A	A
Goal d: The patient does not have nausea Verbalised by patient if conscious	A	A	A	A	A	A
Goal e: The patient is not vomiting	A	A	A	A	A	A
Goal f: The patient is not breathless Verbalised by patient if conscious, consider positional change. Use of a fan may be helpful	A	A	A	A	A	A
Goal g: The patient does not have urinary problems Use of pads, urinary catheter as required	A	A	A	A	A	A
Goal h: The patient does not have bowel problems Monitor – constipation / diarrhoea. Monitor skin integrity Bowels last opened: 7.04.10	A	A	A	A	A	A
Goal i: The patient does not have other symptoms Record symptom here **Pruritus** *If no other symptoms present please record N/A*	A	A	A	A	A	A
Goal j: The patient's comfort & safety regarding the administration of medication is maintained If CSCI in place – monitoring sheet in progress S/C butterfly in place if needed for prn medication location:................................. The patient is only receiving medication that is beneficial at this time. *If no medication required please record N/A*	A	A	A	A	A	A

Name **Karen Jackson**   NHS no **9998887777**   Date **07.04.10**

Section 2   Ongoing assessment of the plan of care – LCP DAY 3 continued

Codes to be recorded at each timed assessment (a moment in time) A= Achieved   V = Variance (exception reporting)

	0400	0800	1200	1600	2000	2400
Goal k: The patient receives fluids to support their individual needs The patient is supported to take oral fluids / thickened fluids for as long as tolerated. Monitor for signs of aspiration and/or distress. If symptomatically dehydrated & not deemed futile, consider clinically assisted (artificial) hydration if in the patient's best interest. If in place monitor & review rate/volume. Explain the plan of care with the patient and relative or carer	A	A	A	A	A	A
Goal l: The patient's mouth is moist and clean See mouth care policy. Relative or carer involved in care giving as appropriate. Mouth care tray at the bedside	A	A	A	A	A	A
Goal m: The patient's skin integrity is maintained Assessment, cleansing, positioning, use of special aids (mattress / bed). The frequency of repositioning should be determined by skin inspection and the patient's individual needs. *Waterlow score:*...................	A	A	A	A	A	A
Goal n: The patient's personal hygiene needs are met Skin care, wash, eye care, change of clothing according to individual needs. Relative or carer involved in care giving as appropriate	A	A	A	A	A	A
Goal o: The patient receives their care in a physical environment adjusted to support their individual needs Well fitting curtains, screens, clean environment, sufficient space at bedside, consider fragrance, silence, music, light, dark, pictures, photographs, nurse call bell accessible	A	A	A	A	A	A
Goal p: The patient's psychological well-being is maintained Staff just being at the bedside can be a sign of support and caring. Respectful verbal and non-verbal communication, use of listening skills, information and explanation of care given. Use of touch if appropriate. Spiritual/religious/cultural needs – consider support of the chaplaincy team	A	A	A	A	A	A
Goal q: The well-being of the relative or carer attending the patient is maintained Just being at the bedside can be a sign of support and caring. Consider spiritual/religious/cultural needs, expressions may be unfamiliar to the healthcare professional but normal for the relative or carer – support of chaplaincy team may be helpful. Listen & respond to worries/fears. Age appropriate advice & information to support children/adolescents available to parents or carers. Allow the opportunity to reminisce. Offer a drink	A	A	A	A	A	A
Signature of the person making the assessment	PSullivan	LR	LR	LR	LR	K.Barr
Signature of the registered nurse per shift	**Night** PSullivan	**Early** L. Roberts		**Late** L. Roberts		**Night** K.Barr

LCP generic version 12 – April 2010
© Marie Curie Palliative Care Institute Liverpool (MCPCIL)

Hospital X

Name **Karen Jackson**   NHS no 9998887777

Section 2	Ongoing assessment MDT progress notes	
Date/time	Record significant events/conversations/medical review/visit by other specialist teams e.g. palliative care / second opinion if sought	Signature
6.4.10	WARD ROUND	
08.00	Pt reviewed – pt clearly dying. LCP to continue – Consultant Signed MDT	
	Sheet. Full discussion regarding the use of S/C fluids. All in agreement.	
	S/C fluids not to be recommenced.	*Dr. S Hughes – F2*
6.04.10	Palliative Care Team	
1100 hours	Decisions regarding the use of S/C fluids noted from the ward round.	*M Cooper CNS*
	I reviewed Karen, patient comfortable, met with family, all concerns	*Ext 3014*
	listened to and support given at this time.	
7.04.10	Palliative Care Team	
0900 hours	Visited patient and family – settled. Patient still appears to be dying. We will	*A Price*
	review in the morning unless contacted.	Nurse Specialist ext 3014
7.4.10	WARD ROUND	
10.00	Day 3 full MDT reassessment. Pt reviewed by SPR, Ward Sister, F2	
	continue with the LCP. Discussed with patient's husband – no questions	*Dr. S Hughes – F2*
	at the current time	
8.04.10	Called to room by husband. Karen has died, may she rest in peace (RIP).	
02.00	Priest called as requested.	
	Doctor on call aware.	Kelly Barr (RGN)
8.04.10	Called to the ward by nursing staff at the request Karen's family.	Fr. Michael Williams
0230	I met with Mr. Jackson, prayers said and all support offered.	
	May she rest in peace.	

Name *Karen Jackson*   NHS no 9998887777

Section 2	Ongoing assessment MDT progress notes	
Date / time	Record significant events/conversations/medical review/visit by other specialist teams e.g. palliative care/second opinion if sought	Signature

LCP generic version 12 – April 2010
© Marie Curie Palliative Care Institute Liverpool (MCPCIL)

Hospital X

Name **Karen Jackson**   NHS no **9998887777**   Date **08.04.10**

Section 3	**Care after death**

Verification of death

Time of the patient's death recorded by the healthcare professional in the organisation: **0200 Hours**

Date of patient's death: 8/4/10

Verified by doctor ☑ Verified by senior nurse ☐   Date / time verified: **8/4/10 0245 Hours**

Cause of death....../..

Details of healthcare professional who verified death

Name: **Dr Alan Philips**   Signature: *A. Philips* Bleep No: **4113**

Comments: **Pupils fixed and dilated no response to painful stimuli. No heart signs, no breath sounds. Patient had died, rest in peace (RIP)**

Persons present at time of death: **Husband, and Staff Nurse**

Relative or carer present at time of death: Yes ☑ No ☐   If not present, have the relative or carer been notified Yes ☐ No ☐

Name of person informed:...../................................ Relationship to the patient:.../..

Contact number:...../................................

Is the coroner likely to be involved: Yes ☐ No ☑

Consultant : **Mr. William Harrison** Doctor: **Dr A Smith** Bleep No: **4433** Tel No: **ext 3621**

Patient Care Dignity	**Goal 10: last offices are undertaken according to policy and procedure** Achieved ☑ Variance ☐ The patient is treated with respect and dignity whilst last offices are undertaken Universal precautions & local policy and procedures including infection risk adhered to Spiritual, religious, cultural rituals / needs met Organisational policy followed for the management of ICDs, where appropriate Organisational policy followed for the management & storage of patient's valuables and belongings
Relative or Carer Information	**Goal 11: The relative or carer can express an understanding of what they will need to do next and are given relevant written information** Achieved ☑ Variance ☐ Conversation with relative or carer explaining the next steps Grieving leaflet given Yes ☑ No ☐ DWP1027 (England & Wales) or equivalent is given Yes ☑ No ☐ Information given regarding how and when to contact the bereavement office / general office / funeral director to make an appointment – regarding the death certificate and patient's valuables and belongings where appropriate Wishes regarding tissue/organ donation discussed Discuss as appropriate: viewing the body / the need for a post mortem / the need for removal of cardiac devices / the need for a discussion with the coroner Information given to families on child bereavement services where appropriate – national & local agencies
Organisation Information	**Goal 12.1: The primary health care team / GP is notified of the patient's death** Achieved ☑ Variance ☐ The primary health care team / GP may have known this patient very well and other relatives or carers may be registered with the same GP Telephone or fax the GP practice **Goal 12.2: The patient's death is communicated to appropriate services across the organisation** Achieved ☑ Variance ☐ e.g. Bereavement office / general office / palliative care team / district nursing team / community matron (where appropriate) are informed of the death The patient's death is entered on the organisation's IT system

Healthcare professional signature: Kelly Barr

   Date: 8.04.10   **Time:** 0300 Hours

Please record any variance on the variance sheet overleaf

Section 3   Care after death MDT progress notes *- record any significant issues not reflected above*

Date	

Name **Karen Jackson**   NHS no **9998887777**

Variance analysis sheet for section 2 – ongoing assessment		
What variance occurred & why? **(What was the issue?)**	**Action taken** **(What did you do?)**	**Outcome** **(Did this solve the issue?)**
Goal: Patient in pain **Signature:** Rachel Doyle **Date / Time:** 5/04/10 2400	Repositioned. Extra pillow given. Given 5mg Morphine S/C **Signature:** Rachel Doyle **Date / Time:** 6/04/10 0010	Patient reviewed following PRN analgesia. Comfortable and pain free **Signature:** Rachel Doyle **Date / Time:** 6/04/10 0030
Goal: S/C butterfly for fluids has fallen out **Signature:** Rachel Doyle **Date / Time:** 5/04/10 2400	Discussed with relatives. As patients currently in pain we have decided to review/replace S/C fluids in the morning **Signature:** Rachel Doyle **Date / Time:** 6/04/10 0010	Dry dressing applied. Will ask the ward team to review S/C butterfly/ S/C fluids on ward round in the morning **Signature:** Rachel Doyle **Date / Time:** 6/04/10 0010
Goal: Relatives concerned as no S/C butterfly in situ for fluids and mouth dry **Signature:** Rachel Doyle **Date / Time:** 6/04/10 0400	Mouth care given, relatives reassured **Signature:** Rachel Doyle **Date / Time:** 6/04/10 0400	Mouth moist and clean. Need for S/C fluids to be discussed this morning. **Signature:** Rachel Doyle **Date / Time:** 6/04/10 0415
Goal: Karen became agitated **Signature:** Kelly Barr **Date / Time:** 8.04.10 0115 hours	No obvious cause for being agitated following my assessment. Midazolam 2.5 mgs given s/c. I will review in 20 minutes **Signature:** Kelly Barr **Date / Time:** 8.04.10 0120 hours	Karen reviewed, now settled, and looks peaceful. **Signature:** Kelly Barr **Date / Time:** 8.04.10 0140 hours
Goal: Karen is in pain **Signature:** Kelly Barr **Date / Time:** 8.04.10 0115 hours	Following my assessment, Morphine 5mgs given S/C. I will review in 20 minutes. **Signature:** Kelly Barr **Date / Time:** 8.04.10 0120 hours	Karen reviewed no complaints of pain and looks peaceful. **Signature:** Kelly Barr **Date / Time:** 8.04.10 0140 hours

Name *Karen Jackson*   NHS no *9998887777*

Variance analysis sheet for section 2 – ongoing assessment

What variance occurred & why? (What was the issue?)	Action taken (What did you do?)	Outcome (Did this solve the issue?)
Goal: Signature:............................... Date / Time:...............................	Signature:............................... Date / Time:...............................	Signature:............................... Date / Time:...............................
Goal: Signature:............................... Date / Time:...............................	Signature:............................... Date / Time:...............................	Signature:............................... Date / Time:...............................
Goal: Signature:............................... Date / Time:...............................	Signature:............................... Date / Time:...............................	Signature:............................... Date / Time:...............................
Goal: Signature:............................... Date / Time:...............................	Signature:............................... Date / Time:...............................	Signature:............................... Date / Time:...............................
Goal: Signature:............................... Date / Time:...............................	Signature:............................... Date / Time:...............................	Signature:............................... Date / Time:...............................

SYMPTOM CONTROL ALGORITHMS

Medicines for symptom control will only be given when needed, following an assessment, and at the right time and just enough and no more than is needed to relieve the symptom.

Merseyside and Cheshire Palliative Care Network Audit Group (2009) Standards and Guidelines Fourth Edition.

Remember:

- ❑ Anticipatory prescribing in this manner will ensure that in the last hours or days of life there is no delay in responding to a symptom if it occurs.
- ❑ Review drug/dose/frequency for patients who are elderly, frail, have dementia or renal failure
- ❑ Not all patients who are dying will require a CSCI (continuous subcutaneous infusion)
- ❑ **If symptoms persist contact the Specialist Palliative Care Team on extension 3014 or bleep 1122**

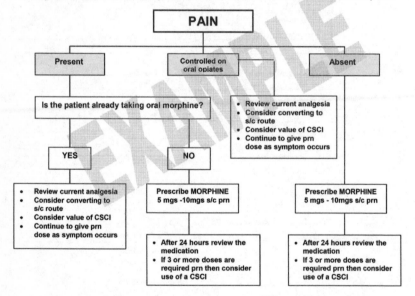

- ➢ **The team is available from 9am – 5pm, 7 days a week.**
- ➢ Out of hours contact number is 0845 666 4444

SUPPORTING INFORMATION

- ❖ To convert from other strong opioids contact the Palliative Care Team / Pharmacy for further advice and support
- ❖ If using opiates for the management of dyspnoea this should be taken into account when titrating opiates for pain
- ❖ Review drug/dose/frequency for patients who are elderly, frail, have dementia or renal failure

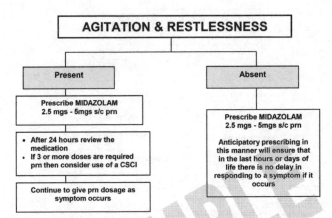

AGITATION & RESTLESSNESS

Present

Prescribe MIDAZOLAM
2.5 mgs - 5mgs s/c prn

- After 24 hours review the medication
- If 3 or more doses are required prn then consider use of a CSCI

Continue to give prn dosage as symptom occurs

Absent

Prescribe MIDAZOLAM
2.5 mgs - 5mgs s/c prn

Anticipatory prescribing in this manner will ensure that in the last hours or days of life there is no delay in responding to a symptom if it occurs

SUPPORTING INFORMATION
- ❖ The management of agitation & restlessness does not usually require the use of opioids unless the agitation & restlessness is thought to be caused by pain
- ❖ Review drug/dose/frequency for patients who are elderly, frail, have dementia or renal failure

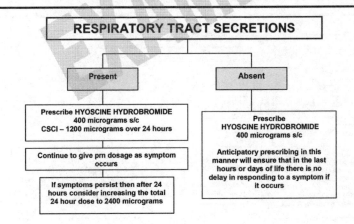

RESPIRATORY TRACT SECRETIONS

Present

Prescribe HYOSCINE HYDROBROMIDE
400 micrograms s/c
CSCI – 1200 micrograms over 24 hours

Continue to give prn dosage as symptom occurs

If symptoms persist then after 24 hours consider increasing the total 24 hour dose to 2400 micrograms

Absent

Prescribe
HYOSCINE HYDROBROMIDE
400 micrograms s/c

Anticipatory prescribing in this manner will ensure that in the last hours or days of life there is no delay in responding to a symptom if it occurs

SUPPORTING INFORMATION
- ❖ Glycopyrronium 200 micrograms s/c prn may be used as an alternative
- ❖ Review drug/dose/frequency for patients who are elderly, frail, have dementia or renal failure

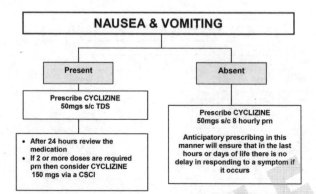

NAUSEA & VOMITING

Present → Prescribe CYCLIZINE 50mgs s/c TDS
- After 24 hours review the medication
- If 2 or more doses are required prn then consider CYCLIZINE 150 mgs via a CSCI

Absent → Prescribe CYCLIZINE 50mgs s/c 8 hourly prn

Anticipatory prescribing in this manner will ensure that in the last hours or days of life there is no delay in responding to a symptom if it occurs

SUPPORTIVE INFORMATION
- ❖ Always use water for the injection when making up Cyclizine.
- ❖ Cyclizine is **NOT** recommended in patients with **heart failure** – seek advice and support
- ❖ Alternative anti-emetics, may be prescribed e.g.
  - ○ HALOPERIDOL 1.5 mgs – 3 mgs s/c prn (1.5 mgs – 5 mgs via a CSCI over 24 hrs – if required)
  - ○ LEVOMEPROMAZINE 6.25 mgs s/c prn (6.25 mgs - 12.5 mgs via CSCI over 24hrs – if required)
- ❖ Review drug/dose/frequency for patients who are elderly, frail, have dementia or renal failure

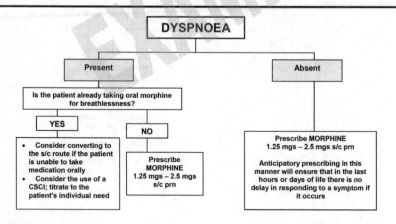

DYSPNOEA

Present → Is the patient already taking oral morphine for breathlessness?

YES
- Consider converting to the s/c route if the patient is unable to take medication orally
- Consider the use of a CSCI; titrate to the patient's individual need

NO
Prescribe MORPHINE 1.25 mgs – 2.5 mgs s/c prn

Absent → Prescribe MORPHINE 1.25 mgs – 2.5 mgs s/c prn

Anticipatory prescribing in this manner will ensure that in the last hours or days of life there is no delay in responding to a symptom if it occurs

SUPPORTIVE INFORMATION
- ❖ If the patient is breathless and anxious, consider Midazolam stat 2.5 mgs s/c prn
- ❖ Review drug/dose/frequency for patients who are elderly, frail, have dementia or renal failure

Appendix 4

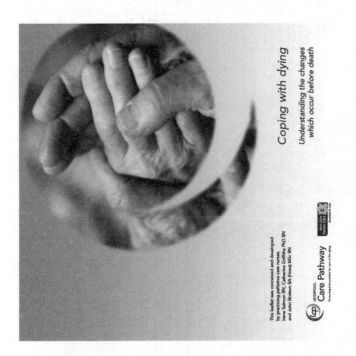

Coping with dying

Understanding the changes which occur before death

This leaflet was conceived and developed by practising palliative care nurses.
Irene Salmon RN, Catherine Griffiths PhD RN and John Bridson BA (Hons) MSc RN

LIVERPOOL
Care Pathway
Promoting best practice for care of the dying

Marie Curie
Cancer Care

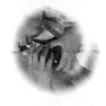

The changes which occur before death

The dying process is unique to each person but in most cases, there are common characteristics or changes which help to indicate that a person is dying.

Any one of these signs can be attributed to something other than dying, so remember that the events to be described here are happening to a person whose illness is already so severe that life is threatened.

The many changes which indicate that life is coming to an end fall into three main categories:

1. Diminished need for food and drink

2. Changes in breathing

3. Withdrawing from the world

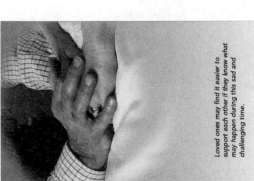

Loved ones may find it easier to support each other if they know what may happen during this sad and challenging time.

There comes a point in most people's lives when death and dying are contemplated. Perhaps we must face our own death or that of someone close to us, but we don't know what to expect.

In order to reduce the anxiety which often comes from the unknown, this leaflet describes some typical features of the process of dying.

It anticipates questions you may want to ask and hopefully it will encourage you to seek further help and information.

Diminished need for food and drink

Initially, as weakness develops, the effort of eating and drinking may simply have become too much and at this time help with feeding might be appreciated.

Your relative/friend will be supported to take food and fluids by mouth for as long as possible.

When someone stops eating and drinking it can be hard to accept, even when we know they are dying. It may be a physical sign that they are not going to get better. Your relative/friend may neither want or need food and/or drink and decisions about the use of artificial fluids (a drip) will be made in the best interests of your relative/friends for this moment in time. This decision will be explained to you and reviewed regularly.

Try not to be discouraged if there is little response – this may be due to weakness, not lack of appreciation. Simply being together can be a great comfort to both of you.

Most importantly, being cared for in this way enables people to feel that their lives have been worthwhile and that they will be remembered.

Changes in breathing

People who suffer from breathlessness are often concerned that they will die fighting for their breath. Yet towards the end of life, as the body becomes less active, the demand for oxygen is actually reduced to a minimum.

This may be comforting to those who have had breathing problems, as carers often remark that when a loved one is dying their breathing is easier than it has been for a long time.

Of course, breathing difficulties can be made worse by feelings of anxiety. But the knowledge that someone is close at hand is not only reassuring; it can be a real help in preventing breathlessness caused by anxiety.

Occasionally in the last hours of life there can be a noisy rattle to the breathing. This is due to a build up of mucus in the chest, which the person is no longer able to cough up. Medication may be used to reduce this and change of position may also help.

These measures may have limited success, but while this noisy breathing is upsetting to carers it doesn't appear to distress the dying person.

If the person is breathing through the mouth, the lips and mouth become dry. Moistening the mouth with a damp sponge and applying lip salve will give comfort.

Withdrawing from the world

Withdrawal from the world is a gradual process. The person will spend more time sleeping and will often be drowsy when awake.

This apparent lack of interest in one's surroundings is part of a natural process which may even be accompanied by feelings of tranquillity. It is certainly not a snub to loved ones.

Eventually the person may lapse into unconsciousness and may remain in this state for a surprisingly long time (in extreme cases many days) although for others it is shorter.

When death is very close (within minutes or hours) the breathing pattern may change again. Sometimes there are long pauses between breaths, or the abdominal muscles (tummy) will take over the work – the abdomen rises and falls instead of the chest. If breathing appears laboured, remember that this is more distressing to you than it is to the person dying.

The skin can become pale and moist and slightly cool prior to death. Most people do not rouse from sleep, but die peacefully, comfortably and quietly.

This is a difficult and painful time for you. You are leaving those you love or losing someone you love and care for. It is often hard to know what to say to each other at a time like this.

Nurses, doctors and other staff are there to help you to work through your worries and concerns and to offer you care and support.

Index